ANATOMY & PHYSIOLOGY FOR
Emergency Care

Workbook

SECOND EDITION

Greg Mullen, MS, NREMT-P

National EMS Academy
South Louisiana Community College
Lafayette, Louisiana

FREDERIC H. MARTINI, PhD
EDWIN F. BARTHOLOMEW, MS
BRYAN E. BLEDSOE, DO, FACEP

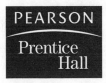

PEARSON

Prentice
Hall

Upper Saddle River, New Jersey 07458

Publisher: Julie Levin Alexander
Publisher's Assistant: Regina Bruno
Senior Acquisitions Editor: Stephen Smith
Associate Editor: Monica Moosang
Editorial Assistant: Patricia Linard
Senior Managing Editor for Development: Lois Berlowitz
Developmental Editor: Allyson Powell
Director of Marketing: Karen Allman
Executive Marketing Manager: Katrin Beacom
Marketing Specialist: Michael Sirinides
Managing Editor for Production: Patrick Walsh
Production Liaison: Faye Gemmellaro
Production Editor: Heather Willison, S4Carlisle
Publishing Services
Manufacturing Manager: Ilene Sanford
Manufacturing Buyer: Pat Brown
Senior Design Coordinator: Christopher Weigand
Cover Designer: Christopher Weigand
Composition: S4Carlisle Publishing Services
Printing and Binding: Bind-Rite Graphics
Cover Printer: Phoenix Color

NOTICE

Our knowledge in clinical sciences is constantly changing. The authors and the publisher of this volume have taken care that the information contained herein is accurate and compatible with the standards generally accepted at the time of the publication. Nevertheless, it is difficult to ensure that all information given is entirely accurate for all circumstances. The authors and the publisher disclaim any liability, loss, or damage incurred as a consequence, directly or indirectly, of the use and application of any of the contents of this volume.

Pearson Prentice Hall™ is a trademark of Pearson Education, Inc.
Pearson® is a registered trademark of Pearson plc
Prentice Hall® is a registered trademark of Pearson Education, Inc.

Pearson Education Ltd.
Pearson Education Singapore, Pte. Ltd.
Pearson Education Canada, Ltd.
Pearson Education—Japan
Pearson Education Australia Pty., Limited

Pearson Education North Asia Ltd.
Pearson Educación de Mexico, S.A. de C.V.
Pearson Education Malaysia, Pte. Ltd.
Pearson Education, Upper Saddle River, New Jersey

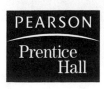

10 9 8 7 6 5 4 3 2 1
ISBN-13: 978-0-13-614021-4
ISBN: 0-13-614021-1

Dedication

To Faith, Dude, Loopy, and Mamel, thanks for the great vacations.
Ellen, how wonderful life is while you're in the world.

Contents

Workbook

Anatomy & Physiology for Emergency Care
SECOND EDITION

INTRODUCTION

Workbook

Anatomy & Physiology for Emergency Care
SECOND EDITION

Welcome to the workbook for *Anatomy & Physiology for Emergency Care*. This workbook has been developed to assist you with the complex world of anatomy and physiology. It can be used as a resource during your anatomy and physiology course or as a self-study guide. The focus of the workbook is to give you the necessary tools to succeed in the class.

This workbook features different styles of test questions that are formatted similar to exam questions used by instructors.

Features

Objectives
The objectives help you reference the content that is covered in *Anatomy & Physiology for Emergency Care*, Second Edition. Page numbers are also provided to make reviewing the material easier.

Exam Questions
Many different exam question styles are used to help assess your mastery of the content from each chapter. We have provided a cross section of these question styles to help you determine your level of understanding of the content. The question styles are:

Multiple Choice: Multiple choice questions are an excellent way to determine your knowledge base in a given area. Multiple choice questions can be written to evaluate your general knowledge of simple to complex topics, which requires you to have an in-depth understanding of a concept or topic. Each chapter has numerous multiple choice questions since that is one of the more common ways you will be tested.

Fill in the Blank: Fill in the blank questions are helpful when evaluating recall information rather than broad concepts or topics. Often these types of questions are used when testing definitions in a certain area.

Ordering: Ordering exercises are helpful when evaluating your knowledge of physiological sequences. This type of exercise allows you to determine the correct sequence of a certain biological function. Only certain select chapters will have this type of evaluation tool.

Matching: Matching exercises are an excellent way to evaluate your understanding of the vocabulary in each chapter. Each chapter has at least 10 matching questions to help you determine your knowledge of the vocabulary from that chapter.

Labeling: Labeling exercises are another way to test your mastery of key anatomy and physiology information presented in the core text. Each workbook chapter contains at least one pertinent labeling exercise.

Short Answer: Short answer questions are usually the type of question that most students dread because this type of question requires a solid understanding of a topic. Most of the other style of exam questions requires you to understand a small portion of a given topic. Short answer questions require you to synthesize numerous ideas or topics and then write the answer in your own words. This type of question is not used often because the answer may be too subjective. But, it is still a good way to determine your knowledge base in a given area.

1 An Introduction to Anatomy and Physiology

Chapter Objectives

1. Describe the basic functions of living organisms.   pp. 3–4

2. Define anatomy and physiology, and describe the various specialties within each discipline.   pp. 4, 5

3. Identify the major levels of organization in living organisms.   p. 5

4. Identify the organ systems of the human body and the major components of each system.   pp. 7–13

5. Explain the significance of homeostasis.   p. 7

6. Describe how negative and positive feedback is involved in homeostatic regulation.   pp. 7, 14–15

7. Use anatomical terms to describe body sections, body regions, and relative positions.   pp. 16–20

8. Identify the major body cavities and their subdivisions.   pp. 20–23

Content Self-Evaluation

MULTIPLE CHOICE

_____ 1. The study of how living organisms perform their vital functions is referred to as _____.
  A. anatomy
  B. physiology
  C. histology
  D. cytology

_____ 2. _____ describes when a stimulus produces a response that opposes the original response.
  A. Positive feedback
  B. Control center
  C. Negative feedback
  D. Homeostasis

_____ 3. _____ describes when a stimulus produces a response that reinforces the original stimulus.
  A. Control center
  B. Negative feedback
  C. Positive feedback
  D. Homeostasis

_____ 4. The _____ plane divides the body into right and left sections.
   A. transverse   C. sagittal
   B. coronal   D. frontal

_____ 5. The _____ plane divides the body into anterior and posterior sections.
   A. transverse   C. sagittal
   B. midsagittal   D. frontal

_____ 6. The thoracic body cavity is subdivided into the _____.
   A. cranial and spinal cavities
   B. abdominal and pelvic cavities
   C. thoracic and abdominal cavities
   D. pleural and pericardial cavities

_____ 7. When utilizing directional references, the term lateral refers to _____.
   A. toward the body's longitudinal axis
   B. away from the body's longitudinal axis
   C. toward an attached base
   D. away from an attached base

_____ 8. When utilizing directional references, the term proximal refers to _____.
   A. toward the body's longitudinal axis
   B. away from the body's longitudinal axis
   C. toward an attached base
   D. away from an attached base

_____ 9. Defense against infection and disease is the major function of which of the following systems?
   A. respiratory system
   B. endocrine system
   C. lymphatic system
   D. integumentary system

_____ 10. Directing long-term changes in the activities of other organ systems is the primary function of which of the following systems?
   A. respiratory system
   B. endocrine system
   C. nervous system
   D. reproductive system

FILL IN THE BLANK

1. _____ is defined as utilizing chemical reactions to provide energy for the body.

2. _____ is the study of the effect of diseases on organ or system functions.

3. The study of cells and their functions is called _____.

4. When studying anatomy and physiology, the word _structure_ relates to the study of _____, while the term _function_ refers to the study of _____.

5. The _____ is the smallest living unit in the body.

6. The _____ system is comprised of organs that are responsible for coordinating the activities of other organ systems.

©2008 Pearson Education, Inc.
Anatomy & Physiology for Emergency Care, 2nd ed.

7. The _____ system stimulates the immune system when needed.

8. The _____ is the part of the respiratory system where gas exchange between air and blood occurs.

9. A simple definition for _____ is a steady state in which the body works most optimally.

10. The diaphragm divides the ventral body cavity into the _____ and the _____ cavities.

TRUE/FALSE

Indicate whether each statement is true or false. Assume that, in all cases, the body is in the anatomical position.

1. The mouth is superior to the nose. _____

2. The trachea is lateral to the esophagus. _____

3. The knee is distal to the femur. _____

4. The heart is medial to the pleural cavity. _____

5. The kidneys are inferior to the adrenal glands. _____

6. The larynx is superior to the spinal cord. _____

7. The hand is distal to the elbow. _____

8. The liver is lateral to the stomach. _____

9. The diaphragm is superior to the large intestine. _____

10. The urethra is proximal to the ureter. _____

LABELING EXERCISE 1–1

Identify the anatomical landmarks shown in Figure 1–1. Place the corresponding letter on the line next to the appropriate label.

_____ 1. Oris

_____ 2. Axilla

_____ 3. Brachium

_____ 4. Patella

_____ 5. Digits (toes)

_____ 6. Thigh

_____ 7. Mentis

_____ 8. Umbilicus

_____ 9. Leg

_____ 10. Antecubitis

_____ 11. Pubis

_____ 12. Antebrachium

_____ 13. Tarsus

_____ 14. Abdomen

_____ 15. Pollex

_____ 16. Pes

_____ 17. Cervicis

_____ 18. Palm

_____ 19. Ear

_____ 20. Carpus

_____ 21. Pelvis

_____ 22. Nasus

_____ 23. Digits (fingers)

_____ 24. Cheek

_____ 25. Thoracis

_____ 26. Eye

_____ 27. Hallux

_____ 28. Forehead

_____ 29. Groin

_____ 30. Mamma

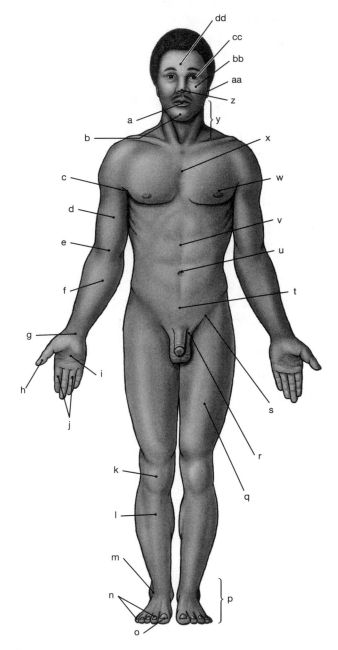

Figure 1–1 Anatomical Landmarks–Anterior View

LABELING EXERCISE 1–2

Identify the anatomical landmarks shown in Figure 1–2. Place the corresponding letter on the line next to the appropriate label.

_____ 1. Dorsum

_____ 2. Popliteus

_____ 3. Planta

_____ 4. Loin

_____ 5. Cephalon

_____ 6. Lower limb

_____ 7. Olecranon

_____ 8. Calcaneus

_____ 9. Cervicis

_____ 10. Calf

_____ 11. Gluteus

_____ 12. Upper limb

_____ 13. Shoulder

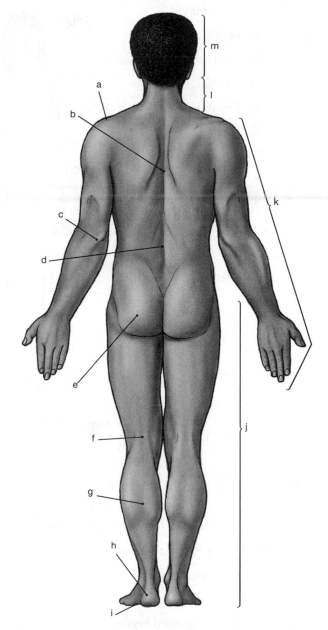

Figure 1–2 Anatomical Landmarks–Posterior View

LABELING EXERCISE 1–3

Identify the directional references in Figure 1–3. Place the corresponding letter on the line next to the appropriate label. _Please use each letter only once._

_____ 1. Proximal

_____ 2. Distal

_____ 3. Inferior

_____ 4. Medial

_____ 5. Caudal

_____ 6. Lateral

_____ 7. Cranial

_____ 8. Proximal

_____ 9. Ventral or anterior

_____ 10. Distal

_____ 11. Superior

_____ 12. Dorsal or posterior

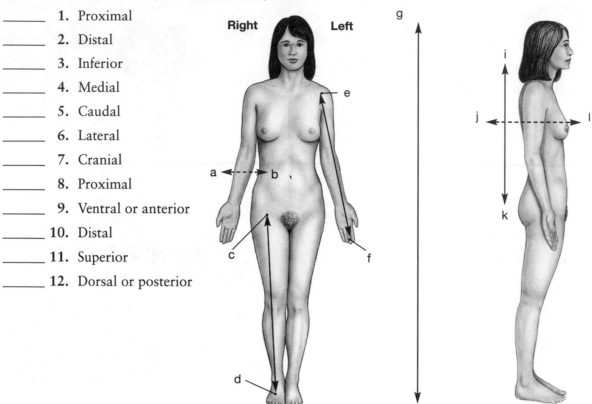

Figure 1–3 Directional References

LABELING EXERCISE 1–4

Identify the abdominopelvic quadrants and regions shown in Figure 1–4. Place the corresponding letter on the line next to the appropriate label.

_____ 1. Right lumbar region

_____ 2. Epigastric region

_____ 3. Left inguinal region

_____ 4. Right inguinal region

_____ 5. Left hypochondriac region

_____ 6. Umbilical region

_____ 7. Hypogastric region

_____ 8. Right hypochondriac region

_____ 9. Left lumbar region

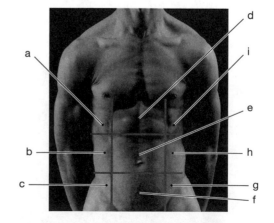

Figure 1–4 Abdominal/Pelvic Quadrants

LABELING EXERCISE 1–5

Identify the parts of the ventral body cavity shown in Figure 1–5. Place the corresponding letter on the line next to the appropriate label.

_____ 1. Diaphragm

_____ 2. Pericardial cavity

_____ 3. Abdominal cavity

_____ 4. Abdominopelvic cavity

_____ 5. Pleural cavity

_____ 6. Peritoneal cavity

_____ 7. Pelvic cavity

_____ 8. Thoracic cavity

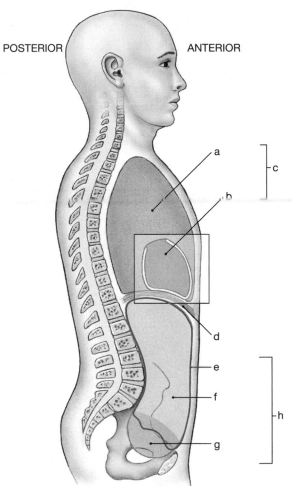

POSTERIOR   ANTERIOR

Figure 1–5 The Ventral Body Cavity

SHORT ANSWER

1. Explain the difference between structure and function as it relates to anatomy and physiology.

_____

_____

_____

2. Provide some examples of how the human body tries to maintain homeostasis in a cold environment.

_____

_____

_____

3. You are called to care for a 10-year-old girl who has twisted her ankle after jumping off a trampoline. You notice significant swelling on the outside of the right ankle and swelling on the inside of the right lower leg about half way up the tibia. Using directional references as a guide, please describe the injury as if you were giving a medical report to a physician.

_____

_____

_____

_____

2 The Chemical Level of Organization

Chapter Objectives

Content Self-Evaluation

MULTIPLE CHOICE

_____ 1. The atomic number represents the number of _____.
   A. protons and neutrons in an atom   C. protons in an atom
   B. neutrons in an atom   D. electrons in an atom

_____ 2. Which of the following is *not* considered a chemical bond?
   A. ionic   C. atomic
   B. covalent   D. hydrogen

_____ 3. Ions with a positive charge are called _____.
   A. electrons   C. anions
   B. cations   D. protons

_____ 4. Which of the following chemical bonds is considered to be the weakest?
A. ionic
B. nonpolar covalent
C. hydrogen
D. polar covalent

_____ 5. Which of the following is *not* true regarding surfactant?
A. lowers surface tension of fluid throughout the lung
B. lines alveoli and smallest bronchioles
C. is produced in the lungs before week 28 gestation of the fetus
D. contains phospholipids and glycoproteins

_____ 6. Which of the following best defines the following reaction?

$$AB \rightarrow A + B$$

A. synthesis reaction
B. exchange reaction
C. decomposition reaction
D. dehydration reaction

_____ 7. The normal human pH range of the blood ranges from _____.
A. 7.00 to 7.35
B. 7.35 to 7.45
C. 7.45 to 7.55
D. 7.00 to 7.15

_____ 8. If the pH in human blood goes below 7.35, the pH is said to be_____.
A. normal
B. acidic
C. alkaline
D. basic

_____ 9. pH is a measurement of the concentration of _____ in a given solution.
A. potassium ions
B. hydroxyl ions
C. hydrogen ions
D. cations

_____ 10. A compound is considered an organic molecule when it contains _____.
A. oxygen and sodium
B. carbon and hydrogen
C. potassium and hydrogen
D. sodium and potassium

_____ 11. Proteins are chains of small organic molecules called _____.
A. lipids
B. amino acids
C. peptides
D. amino group

_____ 12. The most important metabolic fuel in the body is _____.
A. fructose
B. galactose
C. glucose
D. maltose

_____ 13. The most important high-energy compound in the body is _____.
A. RNA
B. DNA
C. ATP
D. H_2O

_____ 14. Which of the following is a disaccharide?
A. fructose
B. glucose
C. sucrose
D. glycogen

_____ 15. A steroid is a _____.
A. lipid
B. carbohydrate
C. protein
D. nucleic acid

FILL IN THE BLANK

1. The formation of table salt (sodium chloride) is an example of a(n) _____ bond.

2. _____ refers to the breakdown of complex molecules within cells.

3. _____ refers to the synthesis of new organic molecules.

4. Enzymes _____ the activation energy needed for a reaction to occur.

5. _____ accelerate chemical reactions in living cells.

6. Carbon dioxide, oxygen, and water are all examples of _____ compounds.

7. The concentration of hydrogen ions in the body is measured by the _____ scale.

8. _____ is an animal starch and is stored in muscle tissues and in the liver.

9. Large carbohydrate molecules are called _____.

10. A fatty acid with double covalent bonds is considered a(n) _____ fatty acid.

11. Peptides are molecules made up of amino acids held together by _____ bonds.

12. The four nitrogen-based molecules that are found in DNA are _____, _____, _____, and _____.

13. The nitrogen-based molecule found only in RNA is _____.

14. ATP is essential for the life of a cell because it provides necessary _____ for the cell to function.

15. ATP is composed of _____ and two phosphate groups.

MATCHING

Match the terms in Column A with the words or phrases in Column B. Write the letter of the corresponding words or phrases in the spaces provided.

Column A

_____ 1. covalent bond

_____ 2. anion

_____ 3. triglycerides

_____ 4. isotopes

_____ 5. enzymes

_____ 6. kinetic energy

_____ 7. lipids

_____ 8. ionic bond

_____ 9. salt

_____ 10. cholesterol

Column B

a. control chemical reactions in the body

b. inorganic compound

c. energy of motion

d. negatively charged ion

e. attraction between two ions

f. consist of three fatty acid molecules

g. atoms that differ in the number of neutrons

h. atoms share electrons to form a molecule

i. precursor of steroid hormones

j. water-insoluble molecules

LABELING EXERCISE 2–1

Identify the points noted on the pH scale shown in Figure 2–1. Place the corresponding letter on the line next to the appropriate label.

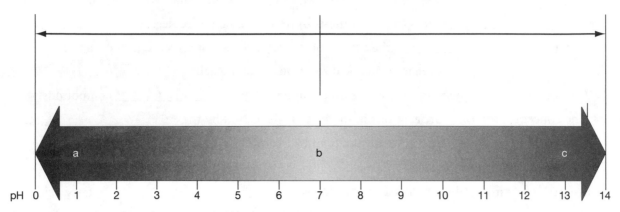

Figure 2–1 pH and Hydrogen Ion Concentration

_____ **1.** Neutral

_____ **2.** Extremely acidic

_____ **3.** Extremely basic

LABELING EXERCISE 2–2

Identify the parts of the nucleic acid shown in Figure 2–2. Place the corresponding letter on the line next to the appropriate label. Please use each letter only once.

_____ **1.** Guanine (G)

_____ **2.** Guanine (G)

_____ **3.** Cytosine (C)

_____ **4.** Adenine (A)

_____ **5.** Adenine (A)

_____ **6.** Thymine (T)

_____ **7.** Thymine (T)

_____ **8.** Adenine (A)

_____ **9.** Guanine (G)

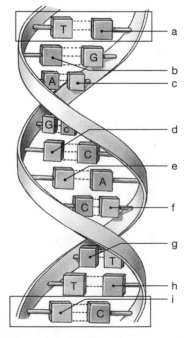

Figure 2–2 The Structure of Nucleic Acids

Short Answer

1. State the differences between hydrolysis and dehydration synthesis.

   _____

   _____

   _____

2. List the four classes of organic compounds found in the body and provide an example of each.

   _____

   _____

   _____

   _____

   _____

3. State the differences between DNA and RNA.

   _____

   _____

   _____

   _____

4. What are the three necessary components that comprise adenosine triphosphate (ATP)?

   _____

   _____

   _____

5. Describe what would occur if the cells of the body stopped producing ATP.

   _____

   _____

   _____

3 Cell Structure and Function

Chapter Objectives

Content Self-Evaluation

MULTIPLE CHOICE

_____ 1. When a cell is selective and only allows certain substances to cross it, the membrane is
            said to be _____.
            A. impermeable   C. selectively permeable
            B. permeable   D. passively permeable

_____ 2. The term *hydrophilic* refers to the cell's ability to react with _____.
            A. fats   C. fatty acids
            B. glycerol   D. water

_____ 3. When a cell shrinks due to a loss of water and a change in osmotic pressure, this is
            referred to as _____.
            A. hemolysis   C. apoptosis
            B. crenation   D. isotonic

_____ 4. The movement of water across a cell membrane occurs by _____.
   A. primary active transport   C. facilitated diffusion
   B. secondary active transport   D. osmosis

_____ 5. Which of the following is true with regard to simple diffusion?
   A. Solute moves from an area of high to low concentration.
   B. Carrier proteins in the cell are required.
   C. It requires energy from ATP.
   D. Solute moves from an area of low to high concentration.

_____ 6. Which of the following is true regarding active transport?
   A. It does not require ATP.
   B. It does not rely on a concentration gradient.
   C. It is used to transport oxygen into the cell.
   D. All of the answer choices are true.

_____ 7. When a red blood cell is placed in contact with a hypotonic solution, the cell will swell and potentially burst. This is referred to as _____.
   A. isotonic   C. crenation
   B. equaltonic   D. hemolysis

_____ 8. IV normal saline (0.9 percent) is considered to be what type of solution?
   A. hypertonic   C. isotonic
   B. hypotonic   D. atonic

_____ 9. Colloid solutions like Dextran or Hetastarch are all considered to be what type of solution?
   A. hypertonic   C. isotonic
   B. hypotonic   D. atonic

_____ 10. The process in which particulate matter is engulfed and brought into the cell is called _____.
   A. phagocytosis   C. exocytosis
   B. pinocytosis   D. repackaging

_____ 11. Which of the following is a simple definition for pinocytosis?
   A. cell eating   C. cell drinking
   B. cell rupture   D. cell excretion

_____ 12. Most of the energy in a cell is produced in the _____.
   A. nucleus   C. mitochondria
   B. cytoplasm   D. Golgi apparatus

_____ 13. Which of the following is one of the functions of the Golgi apparatus?
   A. synthesizes lipids   C. synthesizes proteins
   B. controls metabolism   D. packages and secretes products

_____ 14. Which of the following is a function of the mitochondria?
   A. synthesizes proteins   C. produces ATP
   B. synthesizes lipids   D. controls metabolism

_____ 15. Which of the following is the correct order of steps during mitosis?
   A. metaphase, prophase, telophase, anaphase
   B. prophase, telophase, metaphase, anaphase
   C. prophase, metaphase, anaphase, telophase
   D. prophase, telophase, anaphase, metaphase

©2008 Pearson Education, Inc.
Anatomy & Physiology for Emergency Care, 2nd ed.

FILL IN THE BLANK

1. The smallest functional unit of the body is the _____.

2. The _____ is made up of a phospholipids bilayer.

3. _____ remove damaged organelles or pathogens found in the cell.

4. Lysosomes are produced in the _____.

5. 5 percent dextrose is an example of a(n) _____ solution.

6. During _____ the sodium-potassium pump is necessary to move particles against the concentration gradient.

7. The _____ cell is the only human cell that has a flagellum.

8. The rough endoplasmic reticulum is considered rough due to the presence of _____.

9. A _____ is the functional unit of heredity.

10. Each nucleus contains _____ pair of chromosomes.

11. Transcription of a protein takes place within the _____.

12. The process of mRNA formation is known as _____.

13. The reproduction of male and female sex cells is referred to as _____.

14. The mitotic phase where all of the chromatids line up is _____.

15. Cells in a tumor that no longer respond to control mechanisms are said to be _____.

MATCHING

Match the terms in Column A with the words or phrases in Column B. Write the letter of the corresponding words or phrases in the spaces provided.

Column A

_____ 1. cytoplasm

_____ 2. Golgi apparatus

_____ 3. lysosome

_____ 4. ATP

_____ 5. endoplasmic reticulum

_____ 6. ribosomes

_____ 7. nucleus

_____ 8. centrioles

_____ 9. chromatin

_____ 10. cell membrane

Column B

a. needed for active transport to occur

b. packaging plant of cell

c. digests pathogens

d. synthesize proteins

e. are selectively permeable

f. contains DNA

g. controls metabolism

h. fluid component of cell

i. network of channels in cell

j. play a critical role in cell division

LABELING EXERCISE 3–1

Identify the parts of the cell membrane shown in Figure 3–1. Place the corresponding letter on the line next to the appropriate label. <u>Please use each letter only once</u>.

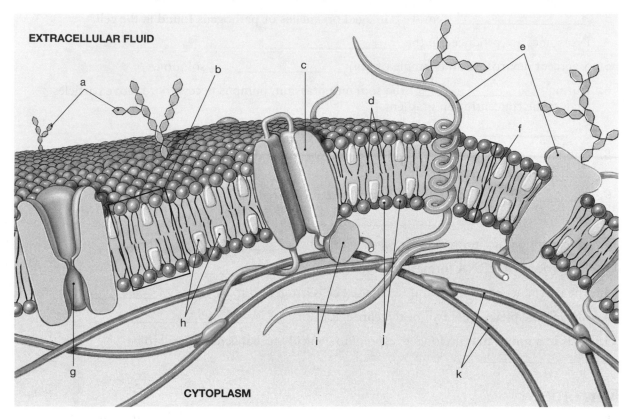

Figure 3–1 The Cell Membrane

_____ **1.** Protein with gated channel

_____ **2.** Carbohydrate chains

_____ **3.** Hydrophobic tails

_____ **4.** Hydrophilic heads

_____ **5.** Cholesterol

_____ **6.** Phospholipid bilayer

_____ **7.** Cytoskeleton

_____ **8.** Proteins

_____ **9.** Protein with channel

_____ **10.** Cell membrane

_____ **11.** Proteins

LABELING EXERCISE 3–2

Identify the parts of the cell shown in Figure 3–2. Place the corresponding letter on the line next to the appropriate label.

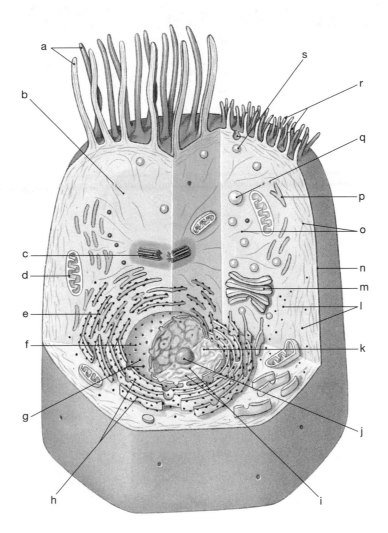

Figure 3–2 The Anatomy of a Cell

_____ 1. Fixed ribosomes

_____ 2. Smooth endoplasmic reticulum

_____ 3. Nuclear envelope surrounding nucleus

_____ 4. Nucleoplasm

_____ 5. Mitochondrion

_____ 6. Golgi apparatus

_____ 7. Cytoskeleton

_____ 8. Lysosome

_____ 9. Cilia

_____ 10. Microvilli

_____ 11. Chromatin

_____ 12. Secretory vesicles

_____ 13. Rough endoplasmic reticulum

_____ 14. Cytosol

_____ 15. Nucleolus

_____ 16. Free ribosomes

_____ 17. Centriole

_____ 18. Cell membrane

_____ 19. Nuclear pores

LABELING EXERCISE 3–3

Identify the steps of cell division shown in Figure 3–3. Place the corresponding letter on the line next to the appropriate label.

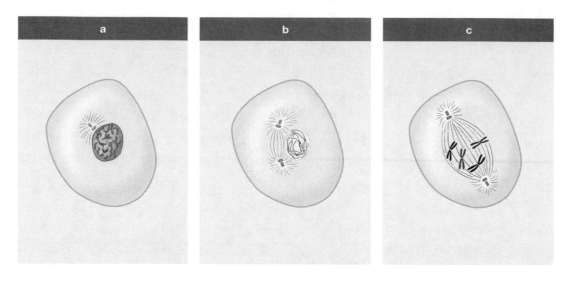

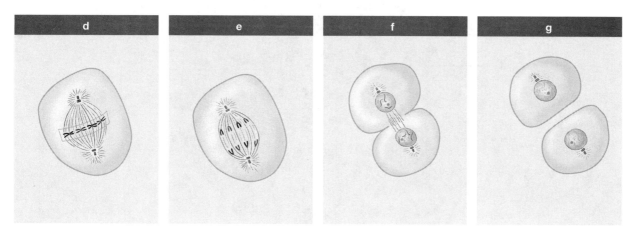

Figure 3–3 Cell Division

_____ 1. Metaphase

_____ 2. Early prophase

_____ 3. Separation

_____ 4. Anaphase

_____ 5. Late prophase

_____ 6. Interphase

_____ 7. Telophase

SHORT ANSWER

1. Describe the general functions of the cell membrane.

   _____

   _____

   _____

   _____

2. Compare the differences between osmosis and diffusion.

   _____

   _____

   _____

   _____

3. What would happen to a red blood cell if you put it into a solution that contains 4.5 percent normal saline?

   _____

   _____

   _____

4. Describe what would happen if during translation of a protein the mRNA codon UAA sequence was presented.

   _____

   _____

   _____

5. What major role will recombinant DNA technology play in the future advancement of medicine?

   _____

   _____

   _____

   _____

4 The Tissue Level of Organization

Chapter Objectives

Content Self-Evaluation

MULTIPLE CHOICE

_____ 1. The four basic types of tissue found in the human body are_____.
  A. skeletal, cardiac, smooth, voluntary
  B. epithelial, muscle, connective, and neural
  C. squamous, cuboidal, columnar, and pseudostratified columnar
  D. cartilage, connective, elastic, adipose

_____ 2. Which of the following is *not* a function of the epithelium?
  A. to provide physical protection   C. to control permeability
  B. to provide insulation   D. to provide sensory information

_____ 3. Which of the following best describes squamous epithelial cells?
   A. hexagonal box-shaped cells   C. flat plate cells
   B. hexagonal narrow or slender cells   D. ciliated cells

_____ 4. In what organ would you expect to find transitional epithelial cells?
   A. small intestine   C. kidney
   B. bladder   D. dermis

_____ 5. Which type of epithelial tissue would you find surrounding kidney tubules?
   A. simple columnar   C. stratified squamous
   B. simple cuboidal   D. pseudostratified columnar

_____ 6. Which of the following is *not* a mechanism by which glandular epithelium releases secretions from glands?
   A. merocrine secretion   C. holocrine secretion
   B. apocrine secretion   D. exocrine secretion

_____ 7. Fat is considered _____ tissue.
   A. dense connective   C. adipose
   B. epithelial   D. columnar

_____ 8. Blood is considered to be what type of tissue?
   A. epithelial   C. squamous
   B. connective   D. adipose

_____ 9. A primary function of adipose tissue is to provide _____.
   A. insulation   C. support
   B. strength   D. conduction

_____ 10. Where are osteocytes located within the structure of the bone?
   A. periosteum   C. lacunae
   B. canaliculi   D. lamella

_____ 11. Which muscle tissue has intercalated discs located within the muscle?
   A. smooth   C. voluntary
   B. skeletal   D. cardiac

_____ 12. Cardiac and skeletal muscle have which of the following similarities?
   A. Both have intercalated discs.
   B. Both are single nucleated muscle cells.
   C. Both are striated.
   D. Both are under voluntary control.

_____ 13. Cardiac and smooth muscle have which of the following similarities?
   A. Both are under voluntary control.
   B. Both are under involuntary control.
   C. Both have intercalated discs.
   D. Both are multinucleated cells.

_____ 14. Which of the following best describes the normal unidirectional flow of an impulse through a neuron?
   A. axon, cell body, dendrite   C. dendrite, cell body, axon
   B. dendrite, axon, cell body   D. cell body, dendrite, axon

_____ 15. Tissue changes that occur with aging can occur because of _____.
   A. hormonal changes   C. lack of proper nutrition
   B. decrease in activity   D. All of the answer choices are correct.

©2008 Pearson Education, Inc.
Anatomy & Physiology for Emergency Care, 2nd ed.

FILL IN THE BLANK

1. _____ glands release secretions directly into tissue or blood.

2. The lipid layers of adjacent cell membranes are tightly bound together by interlocking membrane proteins at a _____.

3. A _____ consists of a single layer of cells that cover the basement membrane.

4. _____ epithelium is found surrounding ducts and kidney tubules.

5. _____ cells are ciliated and are typically found in the respiratory tract.

6. The surface of the skin and the lining of the mouth are comprised of _____ cells.

7. _____ are small, mobile connective tissue cells that migrate into tissues to defend the body against infection.

8. _____ fibers are the most common fibers in connective tissue.

9. _____ syndrome is an inherited connective tissue disease.

10. _____ membranes can be found in the digestive, respiratory, and urinary tracts.

11. _____ tissue can be found between skeletal muscles and helps to reduce friction between muscle.

12. _____ cartilage connects the ribs to the sternum.

13. _____ are the semilunar-shaped cartilages in the knee joint that are often torn during an injury.

14. The axon of one neuron joins the dendrite of another neuron at a specialized site called the _____.

15. An age-related reduction in bone strength in women is known as _____.

MATCHING

Match the terms in Column A with the words or phrases in Column B. Write the letter of the corresponding words or phrases in the spaces provided.

Column A

_____ 1. exocrine gland

_____ 2. squamous epithelium

_____ 3. columnar epithelium

_____ 4. cuboidal epithelium

_____ 5. pseudostratified epithelium

_____ 6. transitional epithelium

_____ 7. chondrocytes

_____ 8. skeletal muscle

_____ 9. smooth muscle

_____ 10. neuron

Column B

a. found in cartilage

b. tall, slender cells

c. secretes onto surface of the skin

d. thin, flat cells

e. found in the bladder

f. often are ciliated

g. found within the kidney tubules

h. muscle with single nucleus

i. conducts electrical impulses

j. multinucleated muscle cell

LABELING EXERCISE 4–1

Several types of tissues are shown in Figure 4–1. Identify the tissue and place the corresponding letter on the line next to the appropriate label on page 27.

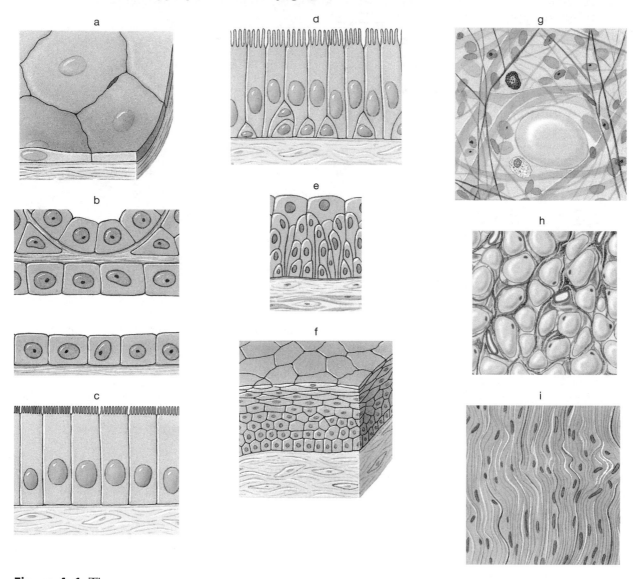

Figure 4–1 Tissues

_____ 1. Simple columnar epithelium

_____ 2. Transitional epithelium

_____ 3. Dense connective tissue

_____ 4. Skeletal muscle tissue

_____ 5. Simple cuboidal epithelium

_____ 6. Hyaline cartilage

_____ 7. Loose connective tissue

_____ 8. Cardiac muscle tissue

_____ 9. Fibrocartilage

_____ 10. Simple squamous epithelium

_____ 11. Bone

_____ 12. Adipose tissue

_____ 13. Elastic cartilage

_____ 14. Stratified squamous epithelium

_____ 15. Smooth muscle tissue

_____ 16. Pseudostratified ciliated
   columnar epithelium

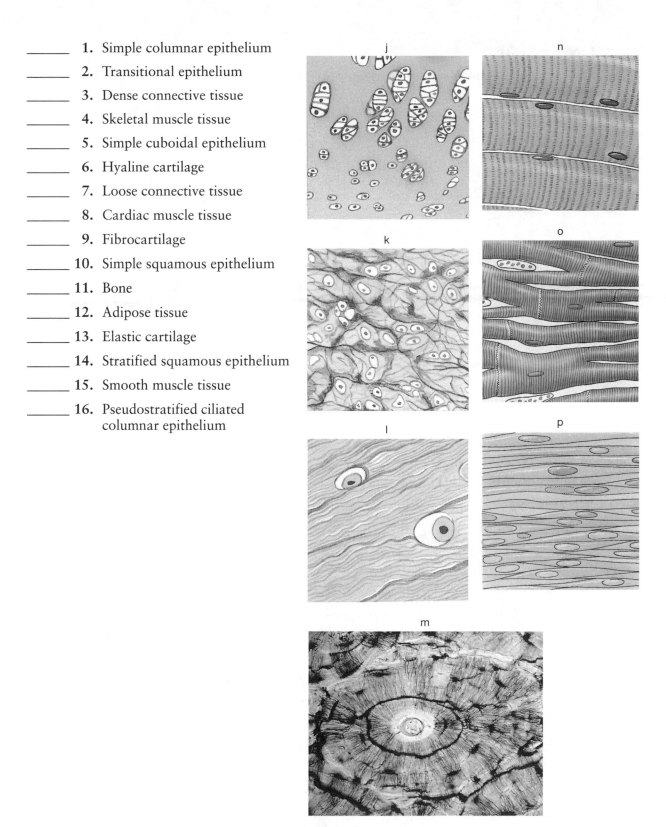

Figure 4–1 _(continued)_

LABELING EXERCISE 4–2

Identify the parts of a neuron shown in Figure 4–2. Place the corresponding letter on the line next to the appropriate label.

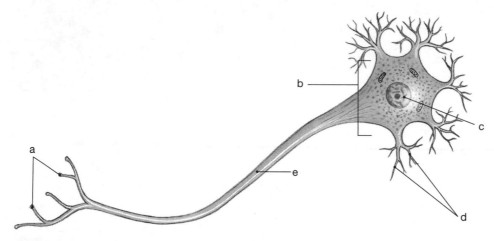

Figure 4–2 A Neuron

_____ 1. Cell body

_____ 2. Dendrites

_____ 3. Axon

_____ 4. Nucleus of neuron

_____ 5. Synaptic terminals

SHORT ANSWER

1. Describe the role macrophages play as a fluid connective tissue.

   _____

   _____

   _____

   _____

2. The ligamentum arteriosum is a ligament that stabilizes the aorta as it descends down from the arch of the aorta. What role may this ligament play in the case of significant blunt trauma to the chest?

   _____

   _____

   _____

   _____

3. Describe the differences between bone and cartilage.

   _____

   _____

   _____

   _____

5 The Integumentary System

Chapter Objectives

Content Self-Evaluation

MULTIPLE CHOICE

_____ 1. Which of the following is *not* a function of the skin?
- A. protection
- B. sensory reception
- C. excretion and secretion
- D. production of vitamin B

_____ 2. Which of the following is the deepest layer of the skin?
- A. stratum corneum
- B. stratum spinosum
- C. stratum germinativum
- D. stratum granulosum

_____ 3. The small muscle attached to the hair is called the _____.
- A. hair papilla
- B. lanugo
- C. hair root
- D. arrector pili

_____ 4. The glands that produce oil to lubricate the skin are called the _____.
- A. endocrine glands
- B. hypocrine glands
- C. sebaceous glands
- D. merocrine glands

_____ 5. Shingles is a viral syndrome that is also referred to as _____.
   A. herpes varicella
   B. herpes zoster
   C. herpes simplex
   D. herpes complex

_____ 6. The outer most layer of the skin is called the _____.
   A. dermis papillae
   B. subcutaneous layer
   C. stratum corneum
   D. stratum germinativum

_____ 7. The layer of skin below the dermis that contains blood vessels is called the _____.
   A. dermal papillae
   B. stratum germinativum
   C. subcutaneous layer
   D. stratum corneum

_____ 8. The layer of the epidermis that undergoes cell replication the most is the _____.
   A. subcutaneous layer
   B. dermal papillae
   C. stratum corneum
   D. stratum germinativum

_____ 9. You are caring for a 30-year-old male with a 3-inch jagged cut on his forearm that looks like it will require sutures. Which of the following best defines this injury?
   A. abrasion
   B. avulsion
   C. laceration
   D. incision

_____ 10. An injury to the skin where a flap of tissue is torn loose or completely off is referred to as a(n) _____.
   A. amputation
   B. abrasion
   C. avulsion
   D. laceration

_____ 11. A _____ burn is sometimes referred to as a partial-thickness burn.
   A. first-degree
   B. second-degree
   C. third-degree
   D. fourth-degree

_____ 12. Which of the following best describes a third-degree burn?
   A. superficial burn with redness
   B. intense pain with limited blistering
   C. damage to all layers of the skin
   D. burn around the mouth and nose area

_____ 13. You are treating an adult burn patient who has sustained second-degree burns to the entire anterior area of the chest and abdomen. What is the total body surface area involved?
   A. 9 percent
   B. 27 percent
   C. 18 percent
   D. 12 percent

_____ 14. You are dispatched to a private home for a 6-year-old child who pulled a pot of boiling water on to himself. You notice numerous blisters and the child is in extreme pain. The burns are best described as _____.
   A. first-degree
   B. second-degree
   C. third-degree
   D. full-thickness

_____ 15. Which of the following is _not_ an age-related change seen in the elderly?
   A. muscles become weaker
   B. increase in macrophages due to increase in infections
   C. sensitivity to the sun increases
   D. sweat glands become less active

©2008 Pearson Education, Inc.
Anatomy & Physiology for Emergency Care, 2nd ed.

FILL IN THE BLANK

1. _____ is an inherited condition caused by a lack of production of melanin from melanocytes.

2. The epidermis contains variable amounts of two pigments, _____ and _____.

3. A small amount of UV radiation stimulates the synthesis of _____.

4. The most common form of skin cancer is _____.

5. A _____ is a secondary lesion that is deep and extends into the dermis.

6. _____ are reddish-purple patches due to blood in the dermis.

7. _____ lubricates the skin and prevents bacterial growth.

8. Sweat glands that secrete their products into hair follicles are called _____.

9. _____ is characterized by dry, itchy patches of skin.

10. A(n) _____ is a simple scrape or scratch on the outer layer of the skin.

11. A(n) _____ may cause massive damage to underlying blood vessels or nerves.

12. A sunburn would be an example of a _____ burn.

13. _____ causes a yellow-orange pigment to appear in the skin. This is commonly seen in newborns.

14. Some medications can be administered through the epidermis. These are called _____ medications.

15. _____ manufacture and store melanin.

MATCHING

Match the terms in Column A with the words or phrases in Column B. Write the letter of the corresponding words or phrases in the spaces provided.

Column A

_____ 1. bilirubin

_____ 2. epidermis

_____ 3. tumor

_____ 4. pustule

_____ 5. ulcer

_____ 6. cyst

_____ 7. full-thickness burn

_____ 8. eczema

_____ 9. partial-thickness burn

_____ 10. laceration

Column B

a. solid lesion

b. loss of epidermis and dermis

c. yellow jaundice

d. encapsulated lesion

e. outermost layer of skin

f. lesion filled with fluid

g. second-degree burn

h. smooth or jagged cut

i. inflammatory skin disease

j. third-degree burn

LABELING EXERCISE 5–1

Identify the parts of the integumentary system shown in Figure 5–1. Place the corresponding letter on the line next to the appropriate label.

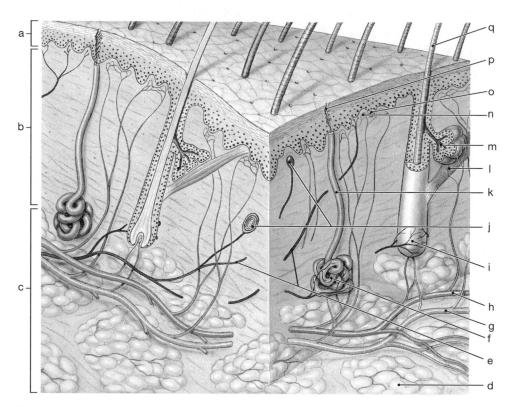

Figure 5–1 The Integumentary System

_____	**1.** Fat		_____	**10.** Artery
_____	**2.** Arrector pili muscle		_____	**11.** Hair shaft
_____	**3.** Dermis		_____	**12.** Sweat gland
_____	**4.** Vein		_____	**13.** Sweat gland duct
_____	**5.** Pore of sweat gland duct		_____	**14.** Subcutaneous layer (hypodermis)
_____	**6.** Sebaceous gland		_____	**15.** Hair follicle
_____	**7.** Epidermis		_____	**16.** Dermal papilla
_____	**8.** Touch and pressure receptors		_____	**17.** Nerve fibers
_____	**9.** Epidermal ridge			

LABELING EXERCISE 5–2

Identify the epidermal layers shown in Figure 5–2. Place the corresponding letter on the line next to the appropriate label.

_____ 1. Stratum lucidum

_____ 2. Stratum germinativum

_____ 3. Stratum spinosum

_____ 4. Basement membrane

_____ 5. Surface

_____ 6. Dermis

_____ 7. Stratum corneum

_____ 8. Epidermis

_____ 9. Stratum granulosum

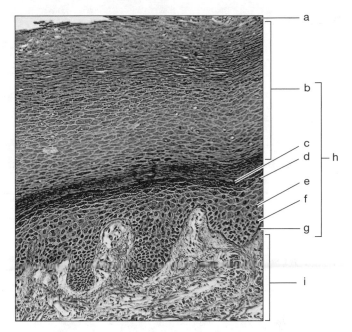

Figure 5–2 The Structure of the Epidermis

LABELING EXERCISE 5–3

Identify the parts of the integumentary system shown in Figure 5–3. Place the corresponding letter on the line next to the appropriate label.

_____ 1. Apocrine duct

_____ 2. Apocrine sweat gland

_____ 3. Dermis

_____ 4. Sweat pore

_____ 5. Arrector pili muscle

_____ 6. Vein

_____ 7. Merocrine sweat gland

_____ 8. Merocrine sweat gland (sectioned)

_____ 9. Hair shaft

_____ 10. Merocrine duct

_____ 11. Epidermis

_____ 12. Artery

_____ 13. Subcutaneous layer

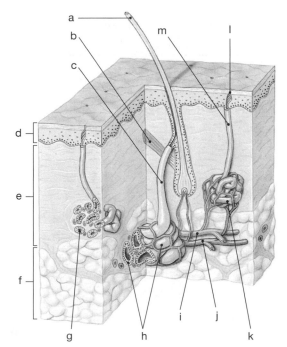

Figure 5–3 Sweat Glands

SHORT ANSWER

1. Discuss how transdermal medications are absorbed through the skin.

   _____

   _____

   _____

   _____

2. Describe the characteristics of a second-degree burn.

   _____

   _____

   _____

3. Discuss the different types of skin cancer and how they occur.

   _____

   _____

   _____

   _____

4. What causes "goose flesh or goose bumps"?

   _____

   _____

   _____

5. What are three functions of the skin?

   _____

   _____

   _____

6 The Skeletal System

Chapter Objectives

Content Self-Evaluation

MULTIPLE CHOICE

_____ 1. Which of the following is *not* a function of the skeletal system?
   A. structural support for the body
   B. storage of calcium and phosphate ions
   C. white blood cell production within the yellow bone marrow
   D. protection of vital organs

_____ 2. The carpal bone is an example of a(n) _____.
   A. short bone   C. flat bone
   B. long bone   D. irregular bone

_____ 3. The humerus is an example of a(n) _____.
   A. short bone   C. flat bone
   B. long bone   D. irregular bone

_____ 4. The vertebrae of the spine are considered _____.
   A. short bones   C. flat bones
   B. long bones   D. irregular bones

_____ 5. The outer surface that covers the bone is called the _____.
   A. diaphysis   C. periosteum
   B. epiphysis   D. endosteum

_____ 6. The central shaft of the bone is called the _____.
   A. metaphysic   C. diaphysis
   B. epiphysis   D. endosteum

_____ 7. Osteocytes can be found within small pockets of the bone called the _____.
   A. lamellae   C. lacunae
   B. canaliculi   D. central canal

_____ 8. A rather new way to provide a route for fluid administration or medications in a life-threatening situation is the intraosseous (IO) route. The IO needle is placed into the _____ of the bone in order to provide emergency fluids or medications.
   A. periosteum   C. medullary cavity
   B. diaphysis   D. osteon

_____ 9. _____ are multinucleated cells that dissolve bony matrix and help regulate calcium concentrations.
   A. Osteocytes   C. Osteoblasts
   B. Osteoclasts   D. Osteons

_____ 10. _____ are responsible for the production of new bone.
   A. Osteocytes   C. Osteoblasts
   B. Osteoclasts   D. Osteons

_____ 11. Rickets is a condition caused by a deficiency in vitamin _____.
   A. A   C. C
   B. B   D. D_3

_____ 12. Which of the following is considered the primary complication of scurvy?
   A. increase in osteoclast production   C. increase in osteoblast production
   B. decrease in osteoclast production   D. decrease in osteoblast production

_____ 13. _____ and _____ are hormones that regulate calcium levels in the body.
   A. Insulin, oxytocin   C. Calcitonin, parathyroid
   B. Oxytocin, thyroxin   D. Calcitonin, thyroid

©2008 Pearson Education, Inc.
Anatomy & Physiology for Emergency Care, 2nd ed.

_____ 14. A ligament attaches _____ to _____.
   A. muscle, muscle
   B. muscle, skin
   C. bone, bone
   D. bone, muscle

_____ 15. Which of the following best categorizes a sprain that causes a complete tear and failure of the ligament?
   A. Grade I
   B. Grade II
   C. Grade III
   D. Grade IV

_____ 16. Which of the following involves a complete displacement of bone ends from a joint?
   A. subluxation
   B. fracture
   C. dislocation
   D. sprain

_____ 17. You have brought in a 7-year-old little boy with an obvious deformity to the proximal tibia. The orthopedic surgeon tells you that it looks like the child has a Salter-Harris fracture that involves the entire epiphysis, and a portion of the metaphysis is broken off. What type of Salter-Harris fracture is this?
   A. Type I
   B. Type II
   C. Type III
   D. Type IV

_____ 18. Which of the following is a type of fracture usually seen in young children?
   A. transverse
   B. comminuted
   C. greenstick
   D. spiral

_____ 19. Which of the following is a type of fracture in which the fracture site has multiple bone fragments?
   A. torus
   B. transverse
   C. oblique
   D. comminuted

_____ 20. At what location in the body may you find a LeFort fracture?
   A. hip
   B. face
   C. shoulder
   D. pelvis

_____ 21. Which group is more at risk for having osteoporosis?
   A. males under 30
   B. females under 30
   C. females over 45
   D. males over 45

_____ 22. The skull is made up of how many bones?
   A. 18
   B. 20
   C. 22
   D. 24

_____ 23. Which of the following is _not_ considered a bone of the skull?
   A. frontal
   B. parietal
   C. occipital
   D. anterior

_____ 24. Which of the following bones does _not_ articulate with any other bone?
   A. lacrimal
   B. hyoid
   C. vomer
   D. zygomatic

_____ 25. There are _____ cervical vertebrae.
   A. 12
   B. 7
   C. 5
   D. 9

_____ 26. The first cervical vertebrae is also called the _____.
   A. dens
   B. axis
   C. atlas
   D. odontoid

_____ 27. The _____ has an S shape and is considered fragile.
   A. scapula
   B. clavicle
   C. radius
   D. ulna

_____ 28. Carpal bones are found in the _____.
  A. foot
  B. ankle
  C. hand
  D. wrist

_____ 29. An immovable joint is referred to as _____.
  A. epithrosis
  B. synarthrosis
  C. amphiarthrosis
  D. diarthrosis

_____ 30. Movement away from the longitudinal axis of the body is referred to as _____.
  A. circumduction
  B. adduction
  C. abduction
  D. hyperextension

FILL IN THE BLANK

1. _____ attach muscle to bone.

2. Mature bone cells are also called _____.

3. _____ are responsible for a process called osteogenesis.

4. The basic functional unit of compact bone is called the _____.

5. _____ dissolve the bony matrix through the process of osteolysis.

6. The growth plate of the bone is also called the _____ plate.

7. Vitamins _____ and _____ are essential for normal bone growth.

8. A _____ fracture is caused by a twisting force to the bone.

9. _____ is a medical condition that leads to weak and brittle bones.

10. The _____ skeleton is the framework that supports and protects vital organ systems.

11. The _____ bone forms part of the floor of the cranium.

12. The _____ articulate with all other facial bones except the mandible.

13. The thoracic region is made up of _____ vertebrae.

14. The thoracic cage is made up of _____ pairs of ribs.

15. At birth, the cranial bones are connected by fibrous tissue known as _____.

16. The pivot joint of the second cervical vertebrae is called the dens or _____.

17. The tip of the sternum is called the _____.

18. The _____ of the ulna is the point of the elbow.

19. The scaphoid bone is found in the _____.

20. The three bones that form the pelvic girdle are the _____, _____ and the _____.

21. The _____ is the longest and heaviest bone in the body.

22. The heel bone is also called the _____.

23. The elbow and knee are examples of _____ joints.

24. A diarthrosis joint is a _____ joint.

25. A pair of fibrocartilage pads called the _____ act as a cushion between the femur and the tibia.

©2008 Pearson Education, Inc.
Anatomy & Physiology for Emergency Care, 2nd ed.

MATCHING

Match the terms in Column A with the words or phrases in Column B. Write the letter of the corresponding words or phrases in the spaces provided.

Group A

Column A

_____ 1. abduction

_____ 2. oblique fracture

_____ 3. transverse fracture

_____ 4. adduction

_____ 5. impacted fracture

_____ 6. segmental fracture

_____ 7. torus fracture

_____ 8. spiral fracture

_____ 9. open fracture

_____ 10. subluxation

Column B

a. partial dislocation

b. skin is broken and communication exists between fracture site and outside environment

c. bone ends at fracture are driven together

d. movement toward the body or toward anatomical position

e. fracture following long axis of the bone

f. buckling of cortex without displacement

g. movement away from the body

h. multiple fracture sites

i. torsion fracture

j. fracture line perpendicular to long axis of the bone

Group B

Column A

_____ 1. shoulder blade

_____ 2. thigh bone

_____ 3. lower leg bone

_____ 4. forearm bone

_____ 5. finger bones

_____ 6. upper arm bone

_____ 7. ankle bones

_____ 8. wrist bones

_____ 9. acetabulum

_____ 10. knee

Column B

a. carpals

b. humerus

c. femur

d. tarsals

e. patella

f. phalanges

g. radius

h. tibia

i. scapula

j. articulates with the head of the femur

LABELING EXERCISE 6–1

Identify the parts of the long bone shown in the Figure 6–1. Place the corresponding letter on the line next to the appropriate label.

_____ 1. Distal epiphysis

_____ 2. Articular cartilage

_____ 3. Compact bone

_____ 4. Spongy bone

_____ 5. Marrow cavity

_____ 6. Proximal epiphysis

_____ 7. Blood vessels

_____ 8. Periosteum

_____ 9. Endosteum

_____ 10. Diaphysis

_____ 11. Epiphyseal line

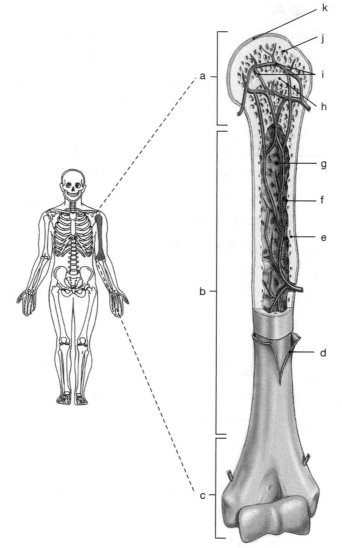

Figure 6–1 The Structure of a Long Bone

©2008 Pearson Education, Inc.
Anatomy & Physiology for Emergency Care, 2nd ed.

LABELING EXERCISE 6–2

Identify the parts of a typical bone shown in Figure 6–2. Place the corresponding letter on the line next to the appropriate label.

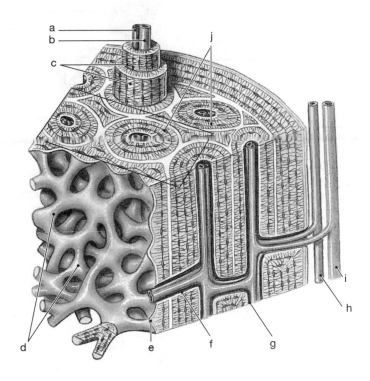

Figure 6–2 The Structure of a Typical Bone

_____ **1.** Perforating canal

_____ **2.** Small vein

_____ **3.** Artery

_____ **4.** Trabeculae of spongy bone

_____ **5.** Osteons

_____ **6.** Capillary

_____ **7.** Vein

_____ **8.** Endosteum

_____ **9.** Lamellae

_____ **10.** Central canal

Identify the axial and appendicular divisions of the skeleton shown in Figure 6–3. Place the corresponding letter on the line next to the appropriate label.

_____ 1. Phalanges

_____ 2. Carpal bones

_____ 3. Clavicle

_____ 4. Tarsal bones

_____ 5. Coxal bone

_____ 6. Sacrum

_____ 7. Phalanges

_____ 8. Rib

_____ 9. Femur

_____ 10. Scapula

_____ 11. Mandible

_____ 12. Parietal bone

_____ 13. Ulna

_____ 14. Fibula

_____ 15. Temporal bone

_____ 16. Metatarsals

_____ 17. Humerus

_____ 18. Maxilla

_____ 19. Metacarpals

_____ 20. Frontal bone

_____ 21. Sternum

_____ 22. Patella

_____ 23. Radius

_____ 24. Tibia

_____ 25. Vertebrae

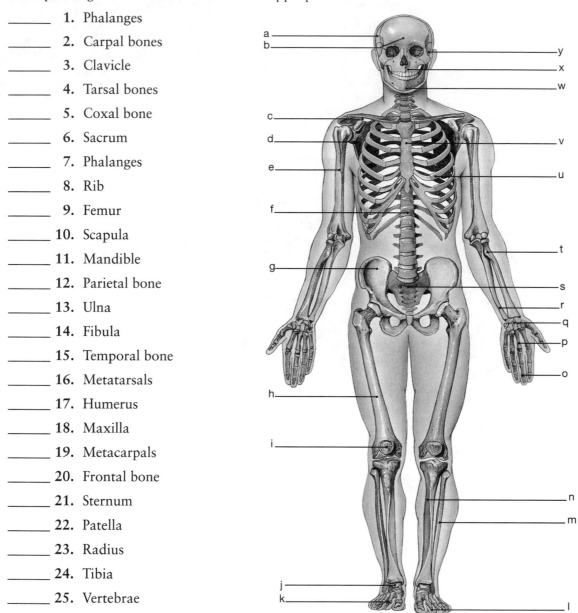

Figure 6–3 The Axial and Appendicular Divisions of the Skeleton

LABELING EXERCISE 6–4

Identify the parts of the adult skull (lateral view) shown in Figure 6–4. Place the corresponding letter on the line next to the appropriate label.

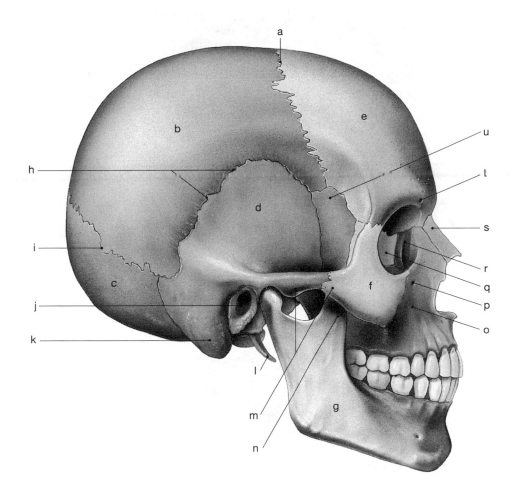

Figure 6–4 The Adult Skull–Lateral View

_____ 1. Styloid process

_____ 2. Coronoid process

_____ 3. External acoustic canal

_____ 4. Squamous suture

_____ 5. Frontal bone

_____ 6. Infraorbital foramen

_____ 7. Occipital bone

_____ 8. Supraorbital foramen

_____ 9. Mandible

_____ 10. Lacrimal bone

_____ 11. Zygomatic bone

_____ 12. Sphenoid bone

_____ 13. Coronal suture

_____ 14. Nasal bone

_____ 15. Ethmoid bone

_____ 16. Lambdoid suture

_____ 17. Maxillary bone

_____ 18. Temporal bone

_____ 19. Zygomatic arch

_____ 20. Parietal bone

_____ 21. Mastoid process

Anatomy & Physiology for Emergency Care, 2nd ed.

LABELING EXERCISE 6–5

Identify the parts of the adult skull (anterior view) shown in Figure 6–5. Place the corresponding letter on the line next to the appropriate label.

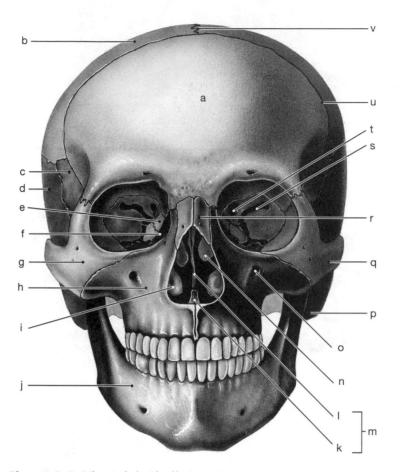

Figure 6–5 The Adult Skull–Anterior View

_____ 1. Perpendicular plate of ethmoid	_____ 12. Inferior nasal concha
_____ 2. Middle nasal concha	_____ 13. Optic canal
_____ 3. Temporal bone	_____ 14. Infraorbital foramen
_____ 4. Mandible	_____ 15. Ethmoid
_____ 5. Mastoid process of temporal bone	_____ 16. Sagittal suture
_____ 6. Maxillary bone	_____ 17. Frontal bone
_____ 7. Superior orbital fissure	_____ 18. Nasal bone
_____ 8. Parietal bone	_____ 19. Bony nasal septum
_____ 9. Lacrimal bone	_____ 20. Zygomatic bone
_____ 10. Temporal process of zygomatic bone	_____ 21. Sphenoid
_____ 11. Coronal suture	_____ 22. Vomer

©2008 Pearson Education, Inc.
Anatomy & Physiology for Emergency Care, 2nd ed.

LABELING EXERCISE 6–6

Identify the parts of the vertebral column shown in Figure 6–6. Place the corresponding letter on the line next to the appropriate label.

_____ 1. Thoracic

_____ 2. Coccygeal

_____ 3. Lumbar

_____ 4. Cervical

_____ 5. Sacral

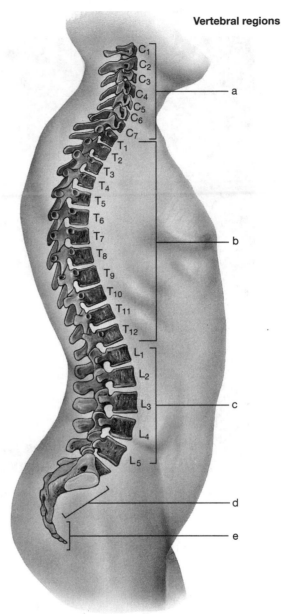

Vertebral regions

Figure 6–6 The Vertebral Column

Identify the parts of the typical vertebrae shown in Figure 6–7. Place the corresponding letter on the line next to the appropriate label.

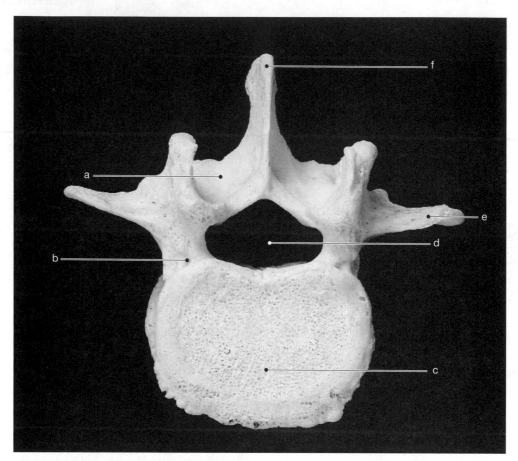

Figure 6–7 Anatomy of a Typical Vertebrae

_____ **1.** Transverse process

_____ **2.** Pedicle

_____ **3.** Vertebral foramen

_____ **4.** Lamina

_____ **5.** Vertebral body

_____ **6.** Spinous process

LABELING EXERCISE 6–8

Identify the parts of the thoracic cage shown in Figure 6–8. Place the corresponding letter on the line next to the appropriate label.

_____ **1.** Costal cartilages

_____ **2.** Sternum

_____ **3.** Floating ribs

_____ **4.** Manubrium

_____ **5.** False ribs

_____ **6.** Body

_____ **7.** True ribs

_____ **8.** Xiphoid process

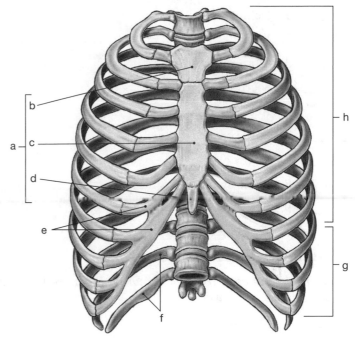

Figure 6–8 Anatomy of the Thoracic Cage

LABELING EXERCISE 6–9

Identify the bones of the wrist and hand shown in Figure 6–9. Place the corresponding letter on the line next to the appropriate label.

_____ **1.** Distal

_____ **2.** Lunate

_____ **3.** Phalanges

_____ **4.** Hamate

_____ **5.** Capitate

_____ **6.** Trapezium

_____ **7.** Triquetrum

_____ **8.** Styloid process of radius

_____ **9.** Trapezoid

_____ **10.** Styloid process of ulna

_____ **11.** Scaphoid

_____ **12.** Metacarpals

_____ **13.** Proximal

_____ **14.** Middle

_____ **15.** Pisiform

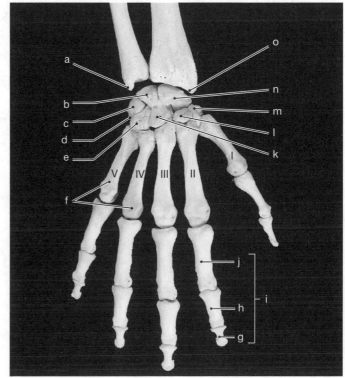

Figure 6–9 Anatomy of the Wrist and Hand

LABELING EXERCISE 6–10

Identify the parts of the pelvis shown in Figure 6–10. Place the corresponding letter on the line next to the appropriate label.

_____ 1. Ischium

_____ 2. Ilium

_____ 3. Obturator foramen

_____ 4. Sacrum

_____ 5. Acetabulum

_____ 6. Pubic crest

_____ 7. Coccyx

_____ 8. Pubic symphysis

_____ 9. Iliac crest

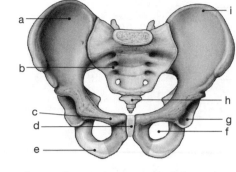

Figure 6–10 Anatomy of the Pelvis

LABELING EXERCISE 6–11

Identify the bones of the foot shown in Figure 6–11. Place the corresponding letter on the line next to the appropriate label.

_____ 1. Phalanges

_____ 2. Tarsal bones

_____ 3. Calcaneus

_____ 4. Navicular

_____ 5. Talus

_____ 6. Cuneiform bone

_____ 7. Tibia

_____ 8. Metatarsal bones

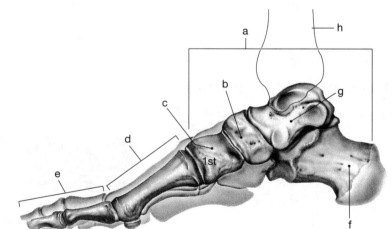

Figure 6–11 Anatomy of the Ankle and Foot

LABELING EXERCISE 6–12

Identify the parts of the knee shown in Figure 6–12. Place the corresponding letter on the line next to the appropriate label. Please use each letter only once.

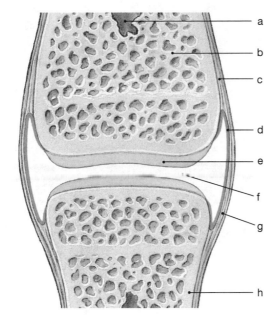

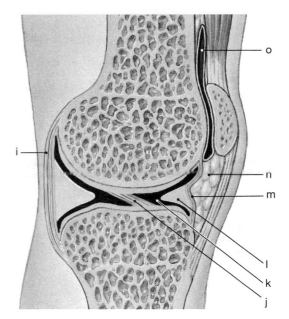

Figure 6–12 The Structure of Synovial Joints

_____ **1.** Intracapsular ligament

_____ **2.** Compact bone

_____ **3.** Articular cartilage

_____ **4.** Meniscus

_____ **5.** Spongy bone

_____ **6.** Fat pad

_____ **7.** Joint capsule

_____ **8.** Bursa

_____ **9.** Joint cavity

_____ **10.** Marrow cavity

_____ **11.** Joint capsule

_____ **12.** Joint cavity (containing synovial fluid)

_____ **13.** Synovial membrane

_____ **14.** Extracapsular ligament

_____ **15.** Periosteum

LABELING EXERCISE 6–13

Identify the parts of the knee joint shown in Figure 6–13. Place the corresponding letter on the line next to the appropriate label.

_____ 1. Medial ligament

_____ 2. Lateral ligament

_____ 3. Medial condyle

_____ 4. Lateral meniscus

_____ 5. Posterior cruciate ligament

_____ 6. Cut tendon

_____ 7. Patellar surface

_____ 8. Fibula

_____ 9. Anterior cruciate ligament

_____ 10. Medial meniscus

_____ 11. Lateral condyle

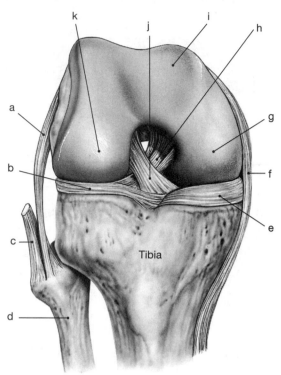

Figure 6–13 Anatomy of the Knee

SHORT ANSWER

1. Discuss the difference between tendons and ligaments.

_____

_____

_____

2. What are the five functions of the skeletal system?

_____

_____

_____

_____

3. Name and give an example of the four types of bone.

_____

_____

_____

4. Describe what could happen to a bone with a damaged epiphyseal plate.

_____

_____

_____

_____

5. What are the four steps of injury and repair that occur to a bone?

_____

_____

_____

_____

_____

7 The Muscular System

Chapter Objectives

Content Self-Evaluation

MULTIPLE CHOICE

_____ 1. Which of the following is *not* a function of the muscular system?
   A. movement of the skeletal system   C. regulate metabolism
   B. maintain posture   D. support soft tissues

_____ 2. Choose the correct order of the typical organization of the skeletal muscle from largest component to smallest.
   A. muscle cells, myofibrils, sarcomere, myofilament
   B. muscle cell, myofilament, sarcomere, myofibril
   C. myofibril, myofilament, muscle cell, sarcomere
   D. myofilament, muscle cell, myofibril, sarcomere

_____ 3. The connective tissue fibers that divide the skeletal muscle into muscle bundles are called the _____.
   A. epimysium   C. endomysium
   B. perimysium   D. mysium

_____ 4. The outermost layer of collagen fibers that surrounds the entire muscle is called the _____.
   A. epimysium   C. endomysium
   B. perimysium   D. fascicle

_____ 5. The _____ surrounds each skeletal muscle fiber.
   A. epimysium   C. endomysium
   B. perimysium   D. fascicle

_____ 6. The _____ is another name for the muscle cell membrane.
   A. sarcomere   C. sarcoplasm
   B. sarcolemma   D. T tubules

_____ 7. A _____ is a bundle of muscle fibers.
   A. fascicle   C. myofibril
   B. T tubule   D. myosin

_____ 8. The boundary that comprises each individual sarcomere is called the _____.
   A. M line   C. A band
   B. Z line   D. I band

_____ 9. Which of the following components of the sarcomere contains the thick filaments?
   A. M line   C. Z line
   B. I band   D. A band

_____ 10. Which of the following ions are responsible for binding to the troponin, which allows for muscle contraction?
   A. sodium   C. magnesium
   B. potassium   D. calcium

_____ 11. Which of the following neurotransmitters is responsible for muscle contraction?
   A. dopamine   C. norepinephrine
   B. serotonin   D. acetylcholine

©2008 Pearson Education, Inc.
Anatomy & Physiology for Emergency Care, 2nd ed.

_____ 12. Striations in muscle can be found in all of the following muscles *except* the _____.
- A. smooth muscle
- B. skeletal muscle
- C. cardiac muscle
- D. All muscles have striations.

_____ 13. Another name for skeletal muscle is _____.
- A. visceral muscle
- B. involuntary muscle
- C. voluntary muscle
- D. smooth muscle

_____ 14. Which of the following statements about acetylcholine (ACh) is correct?
- A. ACh breaks down molecules of cholinesterase.
- B. ACh triggers the contraction of the muscle fiber.
- C. ACh is a product of aerobic metabolism.
- D. ACh changes the permeability of the muscle to calcium.

_____ 15. The point where a nerve connects with a muscle fiber that it is going to stimulate is called the _____.
- A. motor unit
- B. motor neuron
- C. neuromuscular junction
- D. neurotransmitter site

_____ 16. For muscle contraction to stop, which of the following must be present?
- A. acetylcholine
- B. dopamine
- C. acetylcholinesterase
- D. acetylesterase

_____ 17. Which of the following ions rushes into the muscle cell to spread the action potential?
- A. calcium
- B. sodium
- C. potassium
- D. chloride

_____ 18. Calcium ions are released from the _____.
- A. actin
- B. myosin
- C. lysosome
- D. sarcoplasmic reticulum

_____ 19. What could potentially happen if the synapse did not have acetylcholinesterase available?
- A. Muscle would stop contracting.
- B. Muscle would not contract at all.
- C. Muscle would continue contracting.
- D. Acetylcholinesterase has no impact on muscle contraction.

_____ 20. Which of the following is responsible for recharging the energy-spent ADP back to the high-energy ATP?
- A. cAMP
- B. creatine phosphate
- C. glucose
- D. oxygen

_____ 21. After death, the human body becomes stiff from a lack of ATP production. This condition is referred to as _____.
- A. tetanus
- B. myoclonus
- C. paralysis
- D. rigor mortis

_____ 22. An oxygen-containing red pigment that is found within muscle fibers is called _____.
- A. hemoglobin
- B. creatine
- C. globin
- D. myoglobin

_____ 23. Which of the following muscle fibers contains more capillaries and has a greater oxygen supply?
- A. fast fibers
- B. intermediate fibers
- C. slow fibers
- D. white fibers

_____ 24. The muscle in the posterior arm that extends the elbow is the _____.
- A. tricep
- B. bicep
- C. latissimus dorsi
- D. quadriceps

_____ 25. Intercalated discs are found in _____.
   A. visceral muscle   C. skeletal muscle
   B. smooth muscle   D. cardiac muscle

_____ 26. A(n) _____ muscle is the kind of muscle that helps the prime mover work efficiently.
   A. fixator   C. agonist
   B. synergist   D. antagonist

_____ 27. Which of the following is a muscle in the forearm?
   A. triceps   C. deltoid
   B. rhomboid   D. pronator teres

_____ 28. Which of the following is a muscle in the calf?
   A. teres minor   C. gastrocnemius
   B. semitendinosus   D. gracilis

_____ 29. Which of the following is a muscle in the neck?
   A. rhomboid   C. teres major
   B. sartorius   D. sternocleidomastoid

_____ 30. Which of the following muscles would you strengthen by doing sit-ups?
   A. latissimus dorsi   C. rectus abdominis
   B. gluteus minimus   D. soleus

_____ 31. This muscle is attached to the Achilles tendon.
   A. tibialis anterior   C. gracilis
   B. rectus femorus   D. gastrocnemius

_____ 32. When you get thirsty and are drinking a glass of water, this muscle flexes your elbow.
   A. triceps brachii   C. deltoid
   B. biceps brachii   D. latissimus dorsi

_____ 33. You use this muscle when you blow out birthday candles.
   A. frontalis   C. masseter
   B. buccinator   D. pterygoid

_____ 34. The largest superficial muscle that covers the back and portions of the neck is called the _____.
   A. levator scapulae   C. rhomboid
   B. trapezius   D. serratus anterior

_____ 35. Which of the following muscles is *not* part of the quadriceps?
   A. vastus lateralis   C. vastus anterialis
   B. vastus medialis   D. vastus intermedius

ORDERING EXERCISE

Place all of the following steps of the normal skeletal muscle contraction in the correct order using letters A–I.

_____ 1. The binding of acetylcholine at the motor end plate

_____ 2. The active site located on the actin protein is exposed following the binding of calcium (Ca^{2+}) to the troponin complex.

_____ 3. Appearance of the action potential at the sarcolemma

_____ 4. Arrival of an action potential at the synaptic terminal

_____ 5. The cross-bridges detach when the myosin head binds another ATP molecule.

_____ 6. The myosin cross-bridge forms and attaches to the exposed active site on the actin or thin filament.

©2008 Pearson Education, Inc.
Anatomy & Physiology for Emergency Care, 2nd ed.

_____ 7. The detached myosin head is reactivated as it splits the ATP and captures the released energy. The entire cycle is then repeated.

_____ 8. The release of acetylcholine into the synaptic cleft.

_____ 9. The attached myosin head pivots toward the center of the sarcomere, and ADP and a phosphate group are released. This step requires energy stored inside the myosin molecule.

FILL IN THE BLANK

1. _____ are bands of collagen fibers that attach skeletal muscles to bone.

2. The cytoplasm of the muscle is called the _____.

3. Calcium is readily available and found within the _____ of the cell.

4. _____ and _____ are the two contractile proteins that are responsible for muscle contraction.

5. A narrow space called the _____ separates the synaptic terminal from the sarcolemma.

6. _____ is a medical condition that causes the urine to turn a dark reddish color and can cause kidney failure.

7. The thin filaments of the skeletal muscle are covered by strands of a protein called _____.

8. _____ is removed by troponin and calcium prior to muscle contraction.

9. The presence of the molecule ATP is essential for the release of the cross-bridges of the muscle to allow for muscular _____.

10. The toxin _____ prevents the release of acetylcholine and may lead to paralysis.

11. The enzyme _____ may be released during muscle damage or injury.

12. _____ is the most commonly used neuromuscular blocking agent for rapid sequence intubation.

13. Where a muscle begins is referred to as the _____.

14. The muscle that allows you to raise your eyebrows is called the _____.

15. The chewing motions are primarily controlled by the _____ muscle.

16. The muscle that separates the thoracic and abdominal cavities is called the _____.

17. The three muscles that comprise the hamstring are the _____, _____ and the _____.

18. In the elderly, skeletal muscle fibers become _____.

19. Inflammation of the sheath that surrounds the flexor tendons of the palm is called _____ syndrome.

20. _____ is a viral disease that destroys the motor neurons and leads to paralysis.

MATCHING

Match the terms in Column A with the words or phrases in Column B. Write the letter of the corresponding words or phrases in the spaces provided.

Group A

Column A

_____ 1. latissimus dorsi

_____ 2. bicep

_____ 3. orbicularis oris

_____ 4. external oblique

_____ 5. trapezius

_____ 6. extensor carpi radialis

_____ 7. gluteus maximus

_____ 8. sartorius

_____ 9. soleus

_____ 10. flexor digitorum longus

Column B

a. extension and abduction at wrist

b. flexion at knee

c. purses lips

d. plantar flexion at ankle

e. flexion at elbow

f. flexion at joints of toes

g. compresses abdomen

h. adduction and rotation at humerus

i. extend or hyperextend neck

j. lateral rotation at hip

Group B

Column A

_____ 1. synergists

_____ 2. antagonist

_____ 3. deltoid

_____ 4. insertion

_____ 5. origin

_____ 6. adductor magnus

_____ 7. fibromyalgia

_____ 8. rectus femoris

_____ 9. abduction

_____ 10. adduction

Column B

a. muscle injured from pulled groin

b. part of the quadriceps muscle

c. muscles that work together for movement

d. muscles that work opposite of other muscles

e. major abductor of the arm

f. movement toward midline of the body

g. movement away from the midline of the body

h. muscle attached to bone with the greatest movement

i. chronic inflammatory disorder of the muscular system

j. muscle attached to a stationary bone

LABELING EXERCISE 7–1

Identify the parts of the skeletal muscle fiber shown in Figure 7–1. Place the corresponding letter on the line next to the appropriate label.

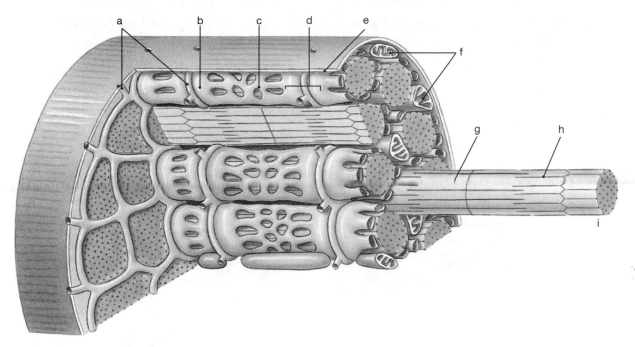

Figure 7–1 A Skeletal Muscle Fiber

_____ 1. T tubules

_____ 2. Mitochondria

_____ 3. Terminal cisterna

_____ 4. Thick filament

_____ 5. Sarcoplasmic reticulum

_____ 6. Thin filament

_____ 7. Triad

_____ 8. Myofibril

_____ 9. Sarcolemma

LABELING EXERCISE 7–2

Identify the steps in skeletal muscle contraction shown in Figure 7–2. Place the corresponding letter on the line next to the appropriate description.

_____ **1.** The cross-bridges detach when the myosin head binds another ATP molecule.

_____ **2.** The detached myosin head is reactivated as it splits the ATP and captures the released energy.

_____ **3.** Resting sarcomere.

_____ **4.** The active site is exposed following the binding of calcium ions to troponin.

_____ **5.** The attached myosin head pivots toward the center of the sarcomere, and ADP and a phosphate group are released.

_____ **6.** The myosin cross-bridge forms and attaches to the exposed active site on the thin filament.

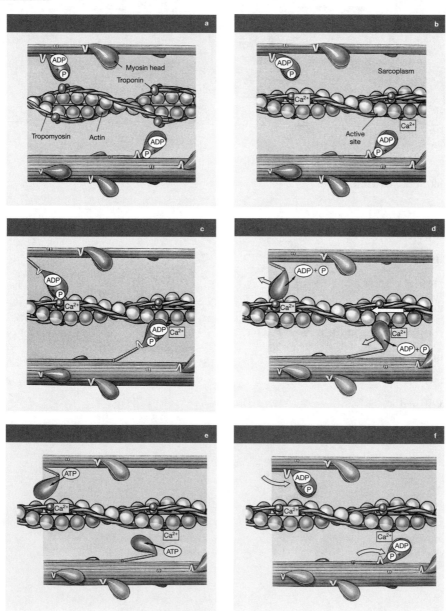

Figure 7–2 The Physiology of Skeletal Muscle Contraction

LABELING EXERCISE 7–3

Identify the major skeletal muscles (anterior view) shown in Figure 7–3. Place the corresponding letter on the line next to the appropriate label.

_____ 1. Flexor carpi ulnaris

_____ 2. Soleus

_____ 3. Extensor carpi radialis

_____ 4. Triceps brachii

_____ 5. Tibialis anterior

_____ 6. Trapezius

_____ 7. Gracilis

_____ 8. Flexor digitorum

_____ 9. Sternum

_____ 10. Pectoralis major

_____ 11. Frontalis

_____ 12. Gastrocnemius

_____ 13. Clavicle

_____ 14. Masseter

_____ 15. Rectus femoris

_____ 16. Serratus anterior

_____ 17. Biceps brachii

_____ 18. External oblique

_____ 19. Palmaris longus

_____ 20. Gluteus medius

_____ 21. Tibia

_____ 22. Temporalis

_____ 23. Pronator teres

_____ 24. Sternocleidomastoid

_____ 25. Vastus medialis

_____ 26. Patella

_____ 27. Latissimus dorsi

_____ 28. Tensor fasciae latae

_____ 29. Rectus abdominis

_____ 30. Brachialis

_____ 31. Brachioradialis

_____ 32. Sartorius

_____ 33. Flexor carpi radialis

_____ 34. Iliopsoas

_____ 35. Extensor digitorum longus

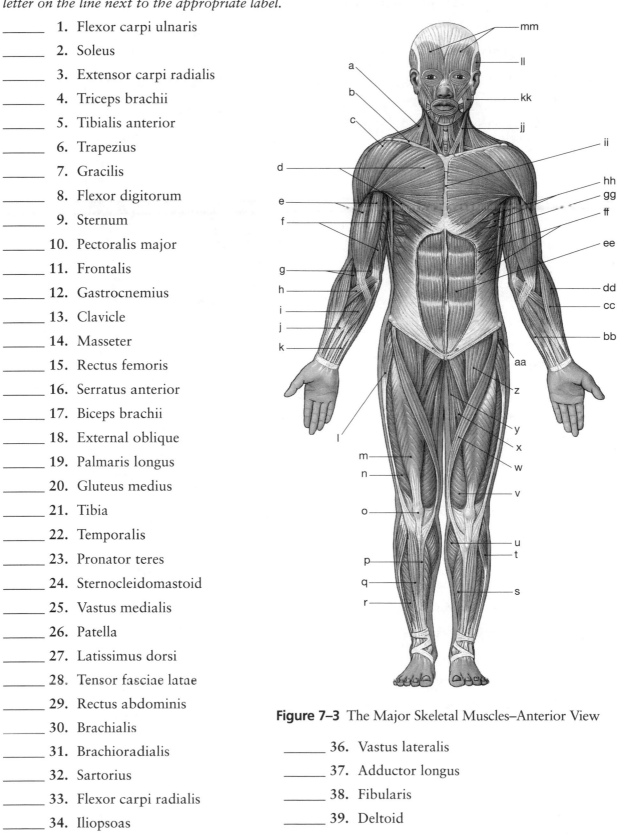

Figure 7–3 The Major Skeletal Muscles–Anterior View

_____ 36. Vastus lateralis

_____ 37. Adductor longus

_____ 38. Fibularis

_____ 39. Deltoid

LABELING EXERCISE 7–4

Identify the major skeletal muscles (posterior view) shown in Figure 7–4. Place the corresponding letter on the line next to the appropriate label.

_____ 1. Semitendinosus

_____ 2. External oblique

_____ 3. Teres minor

_____ 4. Gracilis

_____ 5. Calcaneus

_____ 6. Trapezius

_____ 7. Extensor digitorum

_____ 8. Soleus

_____ 9. Gluteus medius

_____ 10. Teres major

_____ 11. Rhomboid major

_____ 12. Brachioradialis

_____ 13. Occipitalis

_____ 14. Gastrocnemius

_____ 15. Sternocleidomastoid

_____ 16. Adductor magnus

_____ 17. Tensor fasciae latae

_____ 18. Triceps brachii

_____ 19. Biceps femoris

_____ 20. Infraspinatus

_____ 21. Extensor carpi ulnaris

_____ 22. Sartorius

_____ 23. Latissimus dorsi

_____ 24. Flexor carpi ulnaris

_____ 25. Semimembranosus

_____ 26. Extensor carpi radialis

_____ 27. Deltoid

_____ 28. Gluteus maximus

_____ 29. Calcaneal tendon

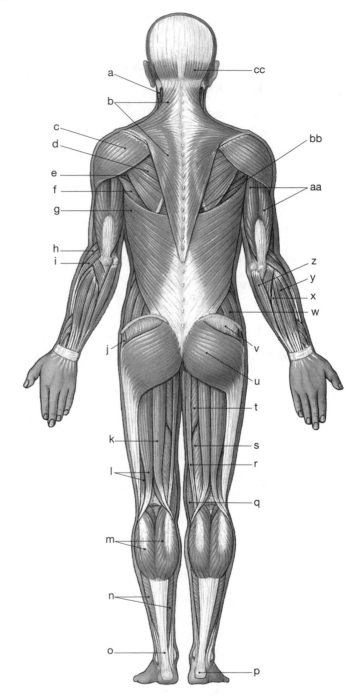

Figure 7–4 The Major Skeletal Muscles–Posterior View

©2008 Pearson Education, Inc.
Anatomy & Physiology for Emergency Care, 2nd ed.

SHORT ANSWER

1. List the three types of muscle tissue and a function for each.

   _____

   _____

   _____

2. Describe what occurs to skeletal muscle during rigor mortis.

   _____

   _____

   _____

3. List the nine steps involved in skeletal muscle contraction. The steps begin with the production of an action potential in the sarcolemma.

   _____

   _____

   _____

   _____

   _____

   _____

   _____

   _____

   _____

   _____

4. Describe what occurs with the medical condition myasthenia gravis.

   _____

   _____

   _____

5. Describe what occurs with the medical condition tetanus.

   _____

   _____

   _____

   _____

8 The Nervous System

Chapter Objectives

Content Self-Evaluation

MULTIPLE CHOICE

_____ 1. The nervous system is comprised of which two divisions?
   A. afferent and efferent
   B. somatic and autonomic
   C. sympathetic and parasympathetic
   D. central and peripheral

_____ 2. The central nervous system is comprised of the _____.
   A. somatic and autonomic divisions
   B. efferent and afferent divisions
   C. brain and spinal cord
   D. visceral and peripheral divisions

_____ 3. Which of the following is *not* a function of the nervous system?
   A. monitors the internal and external environments
   B. integrates sensory information
   C. coordinates voluntary responses from many organ systems
   D. coordinates only involuntary responses of many organ systems

_____ 4. The efferent division of the peripheral nervous system is comprised of which two divisions?
   A. afferent and efferent
   B. sympathetic and parasympathetic
   C. somatic and autonomic
   D. autonomic and afferent

_____ 5. _____ impulses carry information from the peripheral nervous system to the central nervous system.
   A. Efferent
   B. Somatic
   C. Afferent
   D. Autonomic

_____ 6. Which of the following is *not* part of a neuron?
   A. astrocyte
   B. cell body
   C. dendrite
   D. axon

_____ 7. Which of the following gives the gray color to the cell body areas?
   A. axon hillock
   B. collaterals
   C. Nissl bodies
   D. dendrite

_____ 8. Which of the following best describes a bipolar neuron?
   A. two dendrites with a single axon
   B. one dendrite and one axon with a cell body
   C. dendrite and axon are continuous with the cell body
   D. four dendrites with a single axon

_____ 9. Neurons are typically sorted into three functional groups. Which of the following is *not* one of those groups?
   A. interneuron
   B. sensory
   C. motor
   D. collateral

_____ 10. Neurons are classified based on their structure as _____.
   A. motor, sensory, interneurons
   B. multipolar, bipolar, unipolar
   C. afferent, efferent, interneurons
   D. peripheral, central, somatic

_____ 11. The blood-brain barrier is an essential part of isolating the brain from the general circulation. Which one of the following neuroglial cells is responsible for this?
   A. astrocytes
   B. oligodendrocytes
   C. microglia
   D. ependymal

_____ 12. The nodes of Ranvier are part of which neuroglial cell?
   A. astrocyte
   B. oligodendrocyte
   C. microglia
   D. ependymal

©2008 Pearson Education, Inc.
Anatomy & Physiology for Emergency Care, 2nd ed.

_____ 13. Which of the following two neuroglial cells are found in the peripheral nervous system?
A. astrocyte and oligodendrocyte
B. microglial and ependymal
C. Schwann and satellite
D. astrocyte and ependymal

_____ 14. A thin, membranous sheath that increases the speed of the action potential down the axon is called the _____.
A. axon hillock
B. myelin
C. gray matter
D. white matter

_____ 15. All of the following are demyelination disorders _except_ _____.
A. Guillain-Barré syndrome
B. multiple sclerosis
C. muscular dystrophy
D. diphtheria

_____ 16. If the normal resting membrane potential is −70 mV, what would the membrane potential be if the membrane was hyperpolarized?
A. +5 mV
B. −65 mV
C. −80 mV
D. +70 mV

_____ 17. Opening of the sodium channels in the membrane of the neuron results in _____.
A. hyperpolarization
B. repolarization
C. hypopolarization
D. depolarization

_____ 18. Which one of the following ions is responsible for causing the neuron to become hyperpolarized?
A. potassium
B. sodium
C. chloride
D. calcium

_____ 19. Which one of the following neurotoxins can be found in puffer fish?
A. saxitoxin
B. tetrodotoxin
C. ciguatoxin
D. All of the above.

_____ 20. When the action potential of the cell jumps from node to node, it can travel much faster than if traveling through the cell. What is this process called?
A. continuous propagation
B. saltatory propagation
C. depolarization
D. repolarization

_____ 21. Which one of the following ions triggers the release of acetylcholine from the presynaptic membrane?
A. calcium
B. sodium
C. potassium
D. chloride

_____ 22. Organophosphate insecticides like sarin gas have been used in previous terrorist attacks. Which of the following is the principle action of organophosphate poisons?
A. decreases acetylcholine release
B. deactivates acetylcholinesterase
C. increases acetylcholinesterase release
D. deactivates acetylcholine

_____ 23. Which of the following drugs blocks the effects of the organophosphate?
A. epinephrine
B. atropine
C. adrenaline
D. inderal

_____ 24. There are over 50 different known neurotransmitters. Which one of the following neurotransmitters is inhibitory and causes hyperpolarization of the cell?
A. norepinephrine
B. dopamine
C. nitric oxide
D. acetylcholine

_____ 25. Which of the following is the normal order of meningeal layer protection starting from closest to the brain?
A. dura, arachnoid, pia
B. arachnoid, dura, pia
C. dura, pia, arachnoid
D. pia, arachnoid, dura

_____ 26. Bleeding above the dura from a severe head injury is called a _____ hematoma.
   A. subdural
   B. subarachnoid
   C. epidural
   D. epiarachnoid

_____ 27. Which of the following is *not* considered a lobe of the brain?
   A. frontal
   B. anterior
   C. temporal
   D. occipital

_____ 28. The brain stem consists of the _____.
   A. cerebrum, cerebellum, medulla
   B. midbrain, pons, medulla
   C. thalamus, hypothalamus, pons
   D. cerebrum, thalamus, hypothalamus

_____ 29. The primary structure that links the nervous system with the endocrine system is the _____.
   A. medulla
   B. pons
   C. pituitary gland
   D. pineal gland

_____ 30. Which of the following parts of the brain stem is responsible for regulation of heart rate, blood pressure, and respiration?
   A. midbrain
   B. pons
   C. medulla oblongata
   D. cerebellum

_____ 31. The elevated ridges on the outer surface of the brain are called the _____.
   A. sulci
   B. gyri
   C. fissure
   D. lobe

_____ 32. The postcentral gyrus is located in the _____ lobe.
   A. frontal
   B. parietal
   C. occipital
   D. temporal

_____ 33. The speech center of the brain is called (the) _____.
   A. Wernicke's area
   B. Broca's area
   C. prefrontal cortex
   D. hippocampus

_____ 34. If a patient incurred an injury to the hippocampus, which of the following actions would be impacted the most?
   A. walking
   B. talking
   C. memory
   D. speech

_____ 35. Which of the following is *not* a function of the limbic system?
   A. establishing emotional states
   B. linking the conscious intellectual functions of the cerebral cortex with the unconscious and autonomic functions of the brain stem
   C. short-term memory storage and retrieval
   D. long-term memory storage and retrieval

_____ 36. What disease is responsible for damaging the hippocampus and interfering with memory storage?
   A. Parkinson's disease
   B. epilepsy
   C. Alzheimer's disease
   D. seizures

_____ 37. Which one of the following cranial nerves is responsible for controlling the amount of light that enters the eye?
   A. optic
   B. oculomotor
   C. trochlear
   D. abducens

_____ 38. Which cranial nerve is called the wandering nerve?
   A. facial
   B. accessory
   C. vagus
   D. hypoglossal

©2008 Pearson Education, Inc.
Anatomy & Physiology for Emergency Care, 2nd ed.

_____ 39. Which cranial nerve is responsible for hearing?
  A. glossopharyngeal
  B. vestibulocochlear
  C. hypoglossal
  D. trochlear

_____ 40. How many pairs of spinal nerves are there?
  A. 28
  B. 30
  C. 31
  D. 32

_____ 41. A reflex that has a direct connection from the sensory neuron to the motor neuron is referred to as a _____ reflex.
  A. disynaptic
  B. monosynaptic
  C. stretch
  D. flexor

_____ 42. Which of the following divisions of the autonomic nervous system is responsible for the "fight or flight" response?
  A. parasympathetic
  B. sympathetic
  C. cholinergic
  D. ganglionic

_____ 43. Which of the following is *not* a sympathetic nervous system receptor?
  A. alpha
  B. beta
  C. dopamine
  D. gamma

_____ 44. All of the following are common anatomical changes that occur to the brain with age *except* _____.
  A. a reduction in brain size
  B. a reduction in neurons
  C. a decrease in blood flow to the brain
  D. an increase in dendrite branch formation

_____ 45. What percentage of strokes is considered ischemic?
  A. 15 to 20
  B. 40 to 50
  C. 80 to 85
  D. 65 to 70

FILL IN THE BLANK

1. The basic functioning unit of the central nervous system is the _____.

2. Sensory information is transmitted by the _____ division.

3. _____ cells provide a supporting framework for neural tissue.

4. A _____ neuron has two or more dendrites with a single axon.

5. Proprioceptors monitor the _____ and _____ of the skeletal muscles.

6. _____ are responsible for myelination of cells in the central nervous system.

7. _____ is attracted to the negatively charged inner membrane surface of the neuron.

8. When a stimulus triggers a typical action potential, or it does not produce one at all, this is called the _____ principle.

9. A neuron communicates with the muscle cell at the _____.

10. The gaps that are located on the outside of the neuron that allow for the stimulus to travel fast down the axon are called the _____.

11. Acetylcholine is released from the _____ of the neuron.

12. The acetylcholine is broken down in the synapse by an enzyme called _____.

13. The two neurotransmitters of the autonomic nervous system are _____ and _____.

14. The _____ mater is the outermost meningeal layer.

15. The space between the pia and arachnoid mater is called the _____ space.

16. _____ is an infection of the meninges.

17. The end of the spinal cord turns into thread-like extensions called the _____.

18. The cerebrum is divided into two large sections called _____.

19. The _____ contains relay and processing centers for sensory information.

20. Abnormal accumulation of cerebrospinal fluid is called _____.

21. The precentral gyrus can be found in the _____ lobe.

22. _____ is a disorder that affects the ability to speak.

23. _____ refers to a loss of memory from disease or trauma.

24. The hypothalamus is responsible for releasing the hormones _____ and _____.

25. The substantia nigra located within the basal nuclei produces the neurotransmitter _____.

26. The cerebellum helps to maintain _____ and _____.

27. The _____ plexus innervates the shoulder girdle and the upper arm.

28. The two acetylcholine receptors of the parasympathetic nervous system are the _____ and _____.

29. _____ is a progressive disease characterized by the loss of higher cerebral functions.

30. _____ are similar to strokes but the symptoms will spontaneously resolve.

MATCHING

Match the terms in Column A with the words or phrases in Column B. Write the letter of the corresponding words or phrases in the spaces provided.

Group A

Column A	Column B
_____ 1. olfactory	a. vital to autonomic control of visceral function
_____ 2. optic	b. produces facial expressions
_____ 3. oculomotor	c. controls muscles of the tongue
_____ 4. trochlear	d. innervates tongue and pharynx
_____ 5. trigeminal	e. innervates superior oblique muscles of the eye
_____ 6. abducens	f. controls the amount of light into the eye
_____ 7. facial	g. innervates structures in neck and back
_____ 8. vestibulocochlear	h. carry visual information from the eyes
_____ 9. glossopharyngeal	i. monitor sensory receptors of inner ear
_____ 10. vagus	j. responsible for sense of smell
_____ 11. accessory	k. innervates lateral rectus muscle of eye
_____ 12. hypoglossal	l. largest cranial nerve

©2008 Pearson Education, Inc.
Anatomy & Physiology for Emergency Care, 2nd ed.

Group B

Column A

_____ 1. cord concussion

_____ 2. cord compression

_____ 3. complete cord transection

_____ 4. cord hemorrhage

_____ 5. anterior cord syndrome

_____ 6. central cord syndrome

_____ 7. Brown-Séquard syndrome

_____ 8. spinal shock

_____ 9. subdural hematoma

_____ 10. epidural hematoma

Column B

a. complete paralysis below lesion with loss of pain and temperature sensation

b. causes loss of reflexes, bradycardia, and hypotension

c. bleeding above the dura

d. temporary interruption of cord-mediated function

e. results from transection of half of the spinal cord

f. bleeding below the dura

g. results from pressure on the cord causing ischemia

h. causes quadriparesis greater in upper than lower extremities

i. bleeding into neural tissues

j. severing of the spinal cord

LABELING EXERCISE 8–1

Identify the parts of a multipolar neuron shown in Figure 8–1. Place the corresponding letter on the line next to the appropriate label.

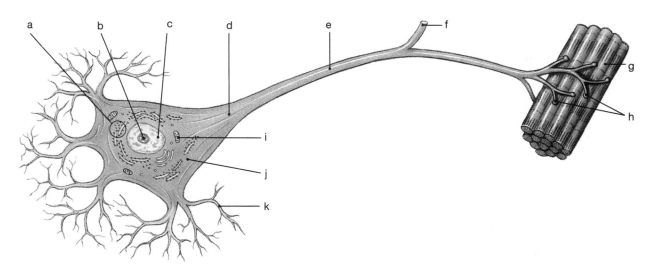

Figure 8–1 Anatomy of a Neuron

_____ 1. Collateral

_____ 2. Nissl bodies

_____ 3. Synaptic terminals

_____ 4. Nucleolus

_____ 5. Skeletal muscle

_____ 6. Nucleus

_____ 7. Mitochondrion

_____ 8. Axon hillock

_____ 9. Dendrite

_____ 10. Axon

_____ 11. Cell body

LABELING EXERCISE 8–2

Identify the major anatomical landmarks on the surface of the left cerebral hemisphere shown in Figure 8–2. Place the corresponding letter on the line next to the appropriate label.

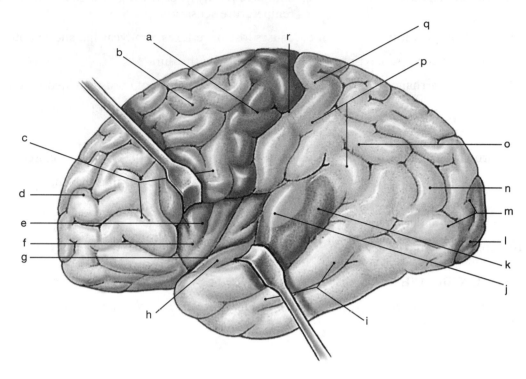

Figure 8–2 The Cerebral Hemisphere

_____ **1.** Auditory cortex

_____ **2.** Visual association area

_____ **3.** Prefrontal cortex

_____ **4.** Olfactory cortex

_____ **5.** Parietal lobe

_____ **6.** Somatic motor association area (premotor cortex)

_____ **7.** Central sulcus

_____ **8.** Lateral sulcus

_____ **9.** Auditory association area

_____ **10.** Insula

_____ **11.** Primary sensory cortex (postcentral gyrus)

_____ **12.** Temporal lobe

_____ **13.** Primary motor cortex (precentral gyrus)

_____ **14.** Visual cortex

_____ **15.** Frontal lobe

_____ **16.** Occipital lobe

_____ **17.** Somatic sensory association area

_____ **18.** Gustatory cortex

LABELING EXERCISE 8–3

Identify the 12 pairs of cranial nerves shown in Figure 8–3. Place the corresponding letter on the line next to the appropriate label.

_____ 1. Abducens

_____ 2. Vagus

_____ 3. Vestibulocochlear

_____ 4. Olfactory

_____ 5. Trochlear

_____ 6. Glossopharyngeal

_____ 7. Optic

_____ 8. Oculomotor

_____ 9. Accessory

_____ 10. Facial

_____ 11. Hypoglossal

_____ 12. Trigeminal

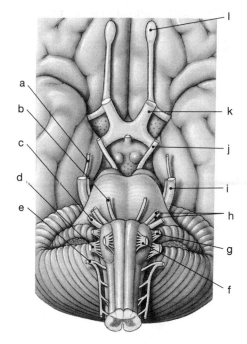

Figure 8–3 The Cranial Nerves

SHORT ANSWER

1. What are the four steps of the neuron action potential? It will begin with the arrival of the action potential at the synaptic knob.

   _____

   _____

   _____

   _____

2. Name two different neurotransmitters, one excitatory and one inhibitory.

   _____

   _____

3. What are the two divisions of the autonomic nervous system? Give examples of the receptors for each.

   _____

   _____

   _____

   _____

   _____

4. List the six major regions of the brain.

_____

_____

5. Describe what a grand mal seizure is.

_____

_____

_____

_____

_____

9 The General and Special Senses

Chapter Objectives

Content Self-Evaluation

MULTIPLE CHOICE

_____ 1. Which of the following is *not* considered a general sense found in the human body?
- A. pain
- B. temperature
- C. pressure
- D. hunger

_____ 2. Which of the following is *not* considered a special sense found in the human body?
- A. hearing
- B. smell
- C. pain
- D. taste

_____ 3. Nociceptors are free nerve endings found on superficial portions of the skin. Nociceptors are sensitive to all of the following stimuli *except* _____.
- A. extreme heat
- B. extreme cold
- C. mechanical damage
- D. chemicals released from injured cells
- E. Nociceptors are sensitive to all of the above.

_____ 4. Which of the following receptors when stimulated will cause analgesia?
   A. mu-2
   B. beta
   C. sigma
   D. epsilon

_____ 5. Which of the following receptors when stimulated will cause hallucinations?
   A. mu-1
   B. mu-2
   C. sigma
   D. kappa

_____ 6. Which of the following nonsteroidal anti-inflammatory medications can be given via intramuscular or intravenous injection?
   A. Tylenol
   B. Motrin
   C. naproxen
   D. Ketorolac

_____ 7. Morphine is commonly used by EMS personnel to treat analgesia. For which of the following receptors does morphine have an affinity?
   A. mu
   B. sigma
   C. beta
   D. epsilon

_____ 8. _____ will not stimulate a mechanoreceptor.
   A. Temperature
   B. Touch
   C. Pressure
   D. Vibration

_____ 9. Which of the following tactile receptors are found in the deepest epidermal layer of the skin and are sensitive to pressure?
   A. Ruffini corpuscles
   B. Meissner's corpuscles
   C. root hair plexus
   D. lamellated corpuscles

_____ 10. Which of the following tactile receptors are sensitive to fine touch and pressure and are found on the eyelids, lips, and fingertips?
   A. Ruffini corpuscles
   B. Meissner's corpuscles
   C. Merkel's discs
   D. lamellated corpuscles

_____ 11. Which of the following tactile receptors are also called pacinian corpuscles?
   A. tactile disc
   B. Merkel's disc
   C. Meissner's corpuscles
   D. lamellated corpuscles

_____ 12. The human body has baroreceptors or pressure receptors that recognize a change in the pressure inside the body. These receptors are located in the _____.
   A. left ventricle
   B. circle of Willis
   C. aortic sinus
   D. jugular veins

_____ 13. Which proprioceptor monitors strain between the tendon and skeletal muscle during muscle contraction?
   A. muscle spindles
   B. Golgi tendon organ
   C. free nerve ending
   D. stretch receptors

_____ 14. Neurons found within the respiratory centers of the brain respond to concentrations of _____ in the cerebrospinal fluid.
   A. oxygen
   B. carbon dioxide
   C. hydroxyl ions
   D. hydrogen ions

_____ 15. The sense of smell is controlled by which of the following cranial nerves?
   A. abducens
   B. olfactory
   C. trigeminal
   D. trochlear

_____ 16. Where are the olfactory receptors located?
  A. back of the throat
  B. sides of the tongue
  C. within the organ of Corti
  D. top of the nasal cavity

_____ 17. The sense of smell is interpreted within the _____.
  A. thalamus
  B. hypothalamus
  C. cerebellum
  D. reticular activating system

_____ 18. The sense of taste is referred to as _____.
  A. olfactory
  B. gastration
  C. gustatory
  D. All of the above.

_____ 19. Specialized epithelial cells and taste receptors form the _____.
  A. papillae
  B. taste pores
  C. gustatory cells
  D. taste buds

_____ 20. Taste buds found within the tongue can differentiate all forms of taste except _____.
  A. sweet
  B. spicy
  C. sour
  D. bitter

_____ 21. Taste buds are monitored by which of the following cranial nerves?
  A. vagus, trigeminal, abducens
  B. glossopharyngeal, vagus, facial
  C. glossopharyngeal, trigeminal, hypoglossal
  D. hypoglossal, glossopharyngeal, vagus

_____ 22. Which of the following cranial nerves assists the olfactory nerve with the perception of "spicy" or "peppery" sensations?
  A. trigeminal
  B. trochlear
  C. vagus
  D. glossopharyngeal

_____ 23. The _____ are considered accessory structures of the eye.
  A. eyelids
  B. superficial epithelium of the eye
  C. structures associated with the production of tears
  D. extrinsic eye muscles
  E. All of the above.

_____ 24. The epithelium that covers the inner surfaces of the eyelids and the outer surface of the eye is called the _____.
  A. sclera
  B. conjunctiva
  C. iris
  D. cornea

_____ 25. The transparent part of the outer layer of the eye is called the _____.
  A. sclera
  B. conjunctiva
  C. iris
  D. cornea

_____ 26. How many different extrinsic eye muscles operate the eye?
  A. two
  B. four
  C. six
  D. eight

_____ 27. The shape of the eye is stabilized in part by the _____.
  A. fibrous tunic
  B. vascular tunic
  C. aqueous humor
  D. vitreous humor

_____ 28. The outermost layer of the eye, which consists of the sclera and cornea, is called the
_____.
A. anterior cavity
B. fibrous tunic
C. vascular tunic
D. neural tunic

_____ 29. Pupillary constriction is controlled by which of the following cranial nerves?
A. optic
B. oculomotor
C. abducens
D. trigeminal

_____ 30. When looking directly at an object, the image that you are looking at falls onto the part
of the retina called the _____.
A. sclera
B. iris
C. fovea centralis
D. cornea

_____ 31. The ability to see in dimly lit rooms or at twilight is controlled by the _____.
A. macula lutea
B. rods
C. cones
D. ganglion cells

_____ 32. The part of the retina that provides sharper, clearer images is called the _____.
A. macula lutea
B. rods
C. cones
D. ganglion cells

_____ 33. The rods and cones are comprised of which type of neuron?
A. unipolar
B. multipolar
C. bipolar
D. ganglion

_____ 34. The optic disc is the origin of which cranial nerve?
A. oculomotor
B. optic
C. abducens
D. trigeminal

_____ 35. A medical condition that leads to an elevated pressure in the eye is called _____.
A. hyphema
B. cataracts
C. conjunctivitis
D. glaucoma

_____ 36. Which of the following is _not_ a name of an auditory ossicle?
A. malleus
B. cochlea
C. incus
D. stapes

_____ 37. The fluid found between the bony and membranous labyrinth is called _____.
A. endolymph
B. perilymph
C. saccule
D. exolymph

_____ 38. The vestibule of the inner ear contains a pair of membranous sacs called the _____.
A. cochlea and cochlear duct
B. semicircular canal and cochlea
C. saccule and utricle
D. tensor and cochlea

_____ 39. The _____ provide(s) information about rotational movements of the head.
A. vestibule
B. semicircular ducts
C. cochlea
D. labyrinth

_____ 40. The receptors of the _____ provide the sense of hearing.
A. vestibule
B. semicircular canals
C. cochlear duct
D. labyrinth

_____ 41. The maculae contain gelatinous material with calcium carbonate crystals called _____.
A. hair cells
B. macular cells
C. otoliths
D. macula

©2008 Pearson Education, Inc.
Anatomy & Physiology for Emergency Care, 2nd ed.

_____ 42. The two vestibular nuclei found at the boundary between the pons and medulla oblongata do all of the following *except* _____.
   A. integrate sensory information arriving from each side of the head
   B. relay information to the cerebellum
   C. relay information to the cerebral cortex
   D. send information to the sensory nuclei within the brain stem and spinal cord

_____ 43. The hair cells of the cochlear duct are located in the _____.
   A. organ of Corti   C. tympanic duct
   B. tectorial membrane   D. basilar membrane

_____ 44. Hearing and equilibrium are controlled through which of the following cranial nerves?
   A. CN VI   C. CN VIII
   B. CN VII   D. CN IX

_____ 45. To help determine hearing loss, a tuning fork is struck and placed near the ear. This is referred to as the _____.
   A. Weber's test   C. Rinne's test
   B. Holmes' test   D. Ménière's test

ORDERING EXERCISE

Place all of the following steps of the physiology of hearing in the correct order using the letters A–F.

_____ 1. The pressure waves distort the basilar membrane on their way to the round window of the tympanic duct.

_____ 2. Sound waves arrive at the tympanic membrane through the external acoustic canal.

_____ 3. Information about the region and intensity of stimulation is relayed to the CNS over the cochlear branch of the vestibulocochlear nerve.

_____ 4. Movement of the tympanic membrane causes displacement of the auditory ossicles.

_____ 5. Vibration of the basilar membrane causes vibration of hair cells against the tectorial membrane and into the organ of Corti.

_____ 6. The movement of the stapes at the oval window establishes pressure waves in the perilymph of the vestibular duct.

FILL IN THE BLANK

1. _____ is a reduction in sensitivity in the presence of a constant stimulus.

2. The perception of pain coming from other parts of the body is called _____.

3. The _____ receptors stimulate respiratory and vasomotor activity.

4. The _____ receptors influence spinal analgesia and sedation.

5. Temperature receptors or _____ are free nerve endings found in the dermis, skeletal muscles, liver, and hypothalamus.

6. Mechanoreceptors are sensitive to stimuli such as _____, _____, and _____.

7. Tactile receptors provide sensations of _____, _____, and _____.

8. An infection in one of the sweat glands between the eyelash follicles produces a painful localized swelling known as a _____.

9. The six extrinsic eye muscles that control the position of the eye are the _____, _____, _____, _____, _____, and the _____.

10. _____ corpuscles are sensitive to pressure and are located in the deepest layer of the dermis.

11. _____ provide information essential to the regulation of autonomic activities by monitoring changes in pressure.

12. _____ sense a change in concentrations of hydrogen ions and carbon dioxide molecules in the cerebrospinal fluid.

13. The sense of smell is provided by paired _____ organs.

14. _____ is an additional taste that has recently been discovered. The taste is characteristic of beef or chicken broth.

15. Glaucoma is a disease caused by a failure of the fluid within the aqueous humor to enter the canal of _____.

16. An _____ is an irregular shape in the lens or cornea that can affect light refraction and clarity of the visual image.

17. The iris attaches to the anterior portion of the _____.

18. Irritation of the conjunctiva is also called _____.

19. The white of the eye is also called the _____.

20. The medical term for unequal pupils is _____.

21. The two types of photoreceptors that are found in the eye are called the _____ and _____.

22. The highest concentration of cones are found in the center of the macula lutea in an area called the _____.

23. The innermost layer of the eye is called the _____.

24. The optic disc does not have photoreceptors, so when light hits in that area you may not see an object. This is called the _____.

25. Blood in the anterior chamber of the eye is called a _____.

26. When the lens of the eye loses its transparency it is called a _____.

27. The process of focusing an image on the retina by changing the shape of the lens is called _____.

28. The medical term for nearsightedness is _____.

29. Visual pigments are derived from the compound _____.

30. All visual pigments are synthesized from vitamin _____.

31. The eardrum is also called the _____ membrane.

32. _____ equilibrium aids us in maintaining our balance when the head and body are moved suddenly.

33. The _____ is the auditory ossicle that attaches to the oval window.

34. The receptors of the inner ear are called _____ cells.

35. _____ equilibrium maintains posture and stability when the body is motionless.

©2008 Pearson Education, Inc.
Anatomy & Physiology for Emergency Care, 2nd ed.

36. Each semicircular duct contains a swollen region called the _____ which contains the sensory receptors.

37. The medical condition for farsightedness in the elderly is called _____.

38. The progressive loss of hearing in the elderly is called _____.

39. The most common cause of blindness in patients over 50 is _____ .

40. Tasting abilities change with age due to the _____.

MATCHING

Match the terms in Column A with the words or phrases in Column B. Write the letter of the corresponding words or phrases in the spaces provided.

Column A

_____ 1. proprioception

_____ 2. nociceptor

_____ 3. substance P

_____ 4. pacinian corpuscles

_____ 5. proprioceptor

_____ 6. olfaction

_____ 7. taste buds

_____ 8. cataract

_____ 9. ultraviolet keratitis

_____ 10. organ of Corti

Column B

a. Golgi tendon organ

b. sense of smell

c. lens loses transparency

d. sense of body position results from this

e. neurotransmitter involved in pain response

f. ocular exposure to tanning lights

g. pain receptor

h. located in cochlear duct

i. taste receptors

j. commonly found on fingers, breast, and genitalia

LABELING EXERCISE 9–1

Identify the parts of the olfactory organs shown in Figure 9–1. Place the corresponding letter on the line next to the appropriate label. <u>Please use each letter only once.</u>

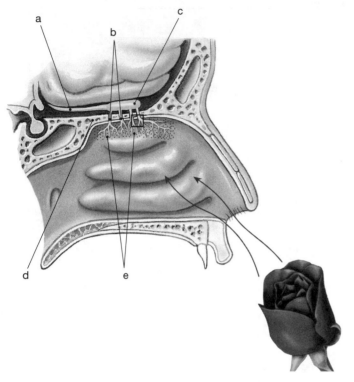

Figure 9–1 The Olfactory Organs

_____	**1.** Cribriform plate of ethmoid		_____	**9.** Olfactory nerve fibers
_____	**2.** Olfactory nerve fibers		_____	**10.** Olfactory cilia
_____	**3.** Olfactory epithelium		_____	**11.** Olfactory tract
_____	**4.** Olfactory receptor cell		_____	**12.** Olfactory bulb
_____	**5.** Regenerative basal cell		_____	**13.** Olfactory gland
_____	**6.** Developing olfactory receptor cell		_____	**14.** Loose connective tissue
_____	**7.** Mucous layer		_____	**15.** Cribriform plate
_____	**8.** Supporting cell		_____	**16.** Olfactory epithelium

LABELING EXERCISE 9–2

Identify the landmarks and features of the eye shown in Figure 9–2. Place the corresponding letter on the line next to the appropriate label.

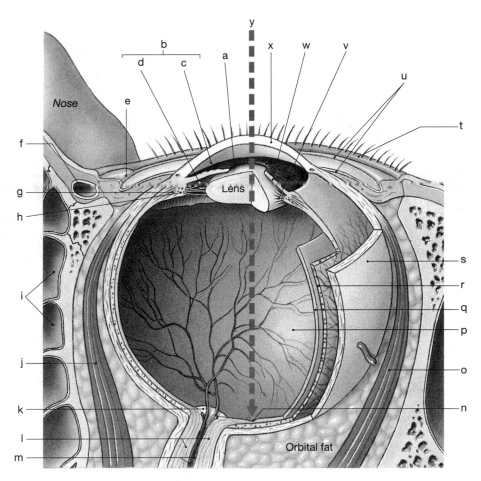

Figure 9–2 Sectional Anatomy of the Eye

_____ **1.** Posterior chamber

_____ **2.** Retina

_____ **3.** Optic disc

_____ **4.** Sclera

_____ **5.** Ciliary muscle

_____ **6.** Medial rectus muscle

_____ **7.** Conjunctiva

_____ **8.** Anterior cavity

_____ **9.** Cornea

_____ **10.** Lacrimal sac

_____ **11.** Lateral rectus muscle

_____ **12.** Visual axis

_____ **13.** Edge of pupil

_____ **14.** Iris

_____ **15.** Central artery and vein

_____ **16.** Lower eyelid

_____ **17.** Anterior chamber

_____ **18.** Choroid

_____ **19.** Ciliary body

_____ **20.** Fovea

_____ **21.** Lacrimal pore

_____ **22.** Posterior cavity (vitreous chamber)

_____ **23.** Ethmoidal sinuses

_____ **24.** Optic nerve

_____ **25.** Suspensory ligament of lens

Identify the parts of the external, middle, and inner ear shown in Figure 9–3. Place the corresponding letter on the line next to the appropriate label.

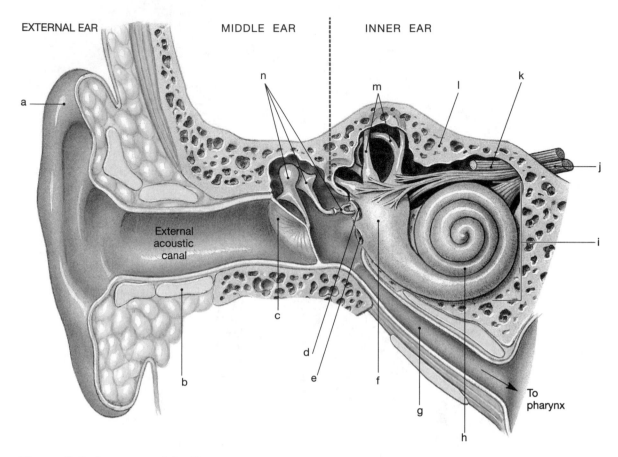

Figure 9–3 Anatomy of the Ear

_____ 1. Vestibule	_____ 8. Cochlea
_____ 2. Semicircular canals	_____ 9. Temporal bone
_____ 3. Cartilage	_____ 10. Auricle
_____ 4. Round window	_____ 11. Facial nerve
_____ 5. Vestibulocochlear nerve	_____ 12. Bony labyrinth of inner ear
_____ 6. Tympanic membrane	_____ 13. Auditory tube
_____ 7. Auditory ossicles	_____ 14. Oval window

LABELING EXERCISE 9–4

Identify the parts of the inner ear shown in Figure 9–4. Place the corresponding letter on the line next to the appropriate label.

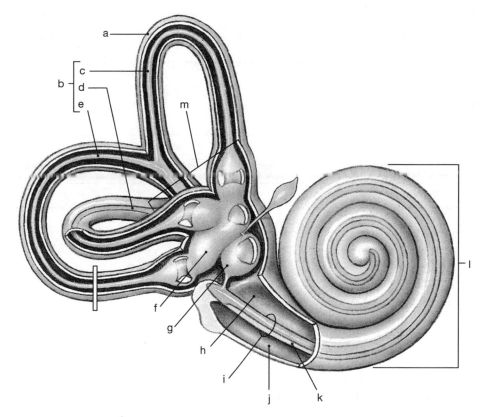

Figure 9–4 Anatomy of the Inner Ear

_____ **1.** Semicircular canal

_____ **2.** Vestibular duct

_____ **3.** Semicircular ducts

_____ **4.** Cochlear duct

_____ **5.** Anterior duct

_____ **6.** Tympanic duct

_____ **7.** Lateral duct

_____ **8.** Organ of Corti

_____ **9.** Posterior duct

_____ **10.** Cochlea

_____ **11.** Utricle

_____ **12.** Vestibule

_____ **13.** Saccule

SHORT ANSWER

1. What are the four kinds of general sense receptors found in the body, and to what stimuli do they respond?

   _____

   _____

   _____

   _____

   _____

2. What are the four primary taste sensations?

   _____

   _____

   _____

   _____

   _____

3. Describe the three layers of the eye.

   _____

   _____

   _____

   _____

   _____

4. Explain what hyphema is and describe its clinical significance.

   _____

   _____

   _____

   _____

5. Describe the pathophysiology of pain pathways and the different medications used to manage pain.

   _____

   _____

   _____

   _____

   _____

   _____

   _____

   _____

   _____

   _____

©2008 Pearson Education, Inc.
Anatomy & Physiology for Emergency Care, 2nd ed.

10 The Endocrine System

Chapter Objectives

Content Self-Evaluation

MULTIPLE CHOICE

_____ 1. Coordination by the nervous and endocrine systems results in:
   A. cellular communication.
   B. release of chemicals that bind to specific receptors.
   C. regulation of negative feedback.
   D. All of the above.

_____ 2. The chemical messengers of the nervous system are called _____, and the chemical messengers of the endocrine system are called _____.
   A. steroids, neurotransmitters
   B. neurotransmitters, hormones
   C. hormones, neurotransmitters
   D. prostaglandins, steroids

_____ 3. Which of the following chemical messengers can be either a hormone or a neurotransmitter?
   A. acetylcholine
   B. epinephrine
   C. insulin
   D. serotonin

_____ 4. All of the following are examples of hormones *except* _____.
   A. melatonin
   B. ADH
   C. oxytocin
   D. acetylcholine

_____ 5. Hormones bind to cell membrane receptors and do not have a direct effect on the cell. Therefore, hormones are considered _____.
   A. first messengers
   B. second messengers
   C. third messengers
   D. fourth messengers

_____ 6. The link between first and second messengers usually involves a _____.
   A. C protein
   B. G protein
   C. A protein
   D. K protein

_____ 7. One of the most important second messengers is _____.
   A. ATP
   B. ADP
   C. cyclic AMP
   D. GTP

_____ 8. Inside the cell, G proteins activate the enzyme adenylate cyclase that converts ATP to _____.
   A. ADP
   B. cyclic AMP
   C. GTP
   D. cyclic GTP

_____ 9. Other examples of second messengers include all of the following *except* _____.
   A. calcium ions
   B. cyclic-GMP
   C. GTP
   D. sodium ions

_____ 10. Free hormones are inactivated when _____.
   A. they diffuse out of the bloodstream and bind to receptors on target cells
   B. they are absorbed and broken down in the liver or kidneys
   C. they are broken down by enzymes in the plasma
   D. All of the above.

_____ 11. Which two hormones are released directly into the circulation at the posterior pituitary gland?
   A. epinephrine and norepinephrine
   B. thyroid and parathyroid
   C. ADH and oxytocin
   D. growth hormone and thyroid hormone

_____ 12. All of the following are functions of the hypothalamus *except* _____.
   A. secretes regulatory hormones that control the activity of the anterior pituitary gland
   B. synthesizes ADH and oxytocin
   C. controls the endocrine cells of the adrenal medullae through sympathetic innervation
   D. releases ADH and oxytocin into the circulation

_____ 13. How many different hormones are released from the pituitary gland?
   A. 7
   B. 9
   C. 11
   D. 13

_____ 14. Regulatory hormone secretion by the hypothalamus is regulated through _____.
   A. negative feedback
   B. positive feedback
   C. cerebellum control
   D. excitatory feedback

_____ 15. Which of the following hormones is *not* released by the anterior pituitary gland?
   A. adrenocorticotropic hormone
   B. anti-diuretic hormone
   C. luteinizing hormone
   D. prolactin

_____ 16. Which of the following hormones targets cells that produce glucocorticoids?
  A. follicle-stimulating hormone
  B. thyroid-stimulating hormone
  C. adrenocorticotropic hormone
  D. growth hormone

_____ 17. Which of the following hormones is responsible for mammary gland development?
  A. follicle-stimulating hormone
  B. luteinizing hormone
  C. growth hormone
  D. prolactin

_____ 18. Which of the following hormones is responsible for inducing ovulation?
  A. follicle-stimulating hormone
  B. luteinizing hormone
  C. prolactin
  D. growth hormone

_____ 19. _____ is responsible for producing testosterone in men.
  A. Follicle-stimulating hormone
  B. Growth hormone
  C. Prolactin
  D. Luteinizing hormone

_____ 20. Patients with diabetes may suffer from polydipsia. Which of the following is the best definition for polydipsia?
  A. decreased urination
  B. increased urination
  C. decreased thirst
  D. increased thirst

_____ 21. Which of the following is the best definition for polyuria?
  A. decreased urination
  B. increased urination
  C. decreased thirst
  D. increased thirst

_____ 22. Which of the following thyroid hormones has three molecules of iodine attached to it?
  A. triiodothyronine
  B. thyroxin
  C. tetraiodothyronine
  D. thyroid-stimulating hormone

_____ 23. C cells of the thyroid gland produce a hormone called calcitonin. Calcitonin helps regulate calcium ion concentration in the body by _____.
  A. inhibiting osteoblasts
  B. inhibiting osteoclasts
  C. increasing osteoclast activity
  D. increasing osteoblast activity

_____ 24. Graves' disease is a disorder of the thyroid gland brought on by _____.
  A. inadequate thyroid hormones in the blood
  B. long-term exposure to inadequate levels of thyroid hormones
  C. prolonged exposure to excess thyroid hormone
  D. excess parathyroid hormone in the blood

_____ 25. Myxedema is a thyroid condition caused by _____.
  A. inadequate thyroid hormones in the blood
  B. long-term exposure to inadequate levels of thyroid hormones
  C. prolonged exposure to excess thyroid hormone
  D. excess parathyroid hormone in the blood

_____ 26. Low calcium concentrations may be dangerous because of an increase in cell permeability to _____. This may lead to an increase in cell excitability and lead to seizures or muscle spasms.
  A. sodium
  B. potassium
  C. chloride
  D. magnesium

_____ 27. All of the following are risk factors for developing thyroid disease _except_ _____.
  A. hypertension
  B. female sex
  C. elderly patient
  D. goiter

_____ 28. In what age group does Graves' disease typically occur?
  A. pediatric
  B. young adult
  C. adult
  D. geriatric

_____ 29. _____ is *not* a sign or symptom of Graves' disease.
   A. Agitation   C. Weakness
   B. Insomnia   D. Weight gain

_____ 30. Which of the following is *not* a sign or symptom of thyrotoxic crisis?
   A. fever   C. bradycardia
   B. tachycardia   D. hypotension

_____ 31. The chief cells in the parathyroid gland monitor which of the following ion concentrations?
   A. sodium   C. calcium
   B. potassium   D. magnesium

_____ 32. Which of the following is true regarding the parathyroid gland?
   A. inhibits osteoclast activity   C. increases urinary excretion of calcium
   B. stimulates osteoblast activity   D. stimulates kidneys to form calcitriol

_____ 33. Which of the following is *not* produced within the adrenal cortex?
   A. aldosterone   C. angiotensin
   B. cortisol   D. androgens

_____ 34. _____ is the corticosteroid that is responsible for the conservation of sodium ions.
   A. Cortisol   C. Aldosterone
   B. Estrogen   D. Hydrocortisone

_____ 35. _____ act as an anti-inflammatory agent.
   A. Glucocorticoids   C. Androgens
   B. Mineralocorticoids D. Estrogens

_____ 36. Which of the following chemicals is secreted from the adrenal medulla the largest percentage of the time?
   A. norepinephrine   C. ATP
   B. epinephrine   D. glycogen

_____ 37. _____ is caused by excessive glucocorticoid release.
   A. Addison's disease C. Diabetes
   B. Graves' disease   D. Cushing's syndrome

_____ 38. Which of the following diseases is caused by a destruction of the adrenal cortex which produces corticosteroids?
   A. Addison's disease C. diabetes
   B. Graves' disease   D. Cushing's syndrome

_____ 39. The pineal gland produces a very important hormone called melatonin. Which of the following are examples of the functions of melatonin?
   A. It slows the maturation of the reproductive organs.
   B. It acts as an antioxidant against free radicals such as hydrogen peroxide and nitric oxide.
   C. It establishes the day/night activity cycle.
   D. All of the above.

_____ 40. One of the main functions of the pancreas is to regulate glucose metabolism. It does so through a group of cells within the pancreas. One group of cells is called alpha cells. They are responsible for producing _____.
   A. glycogen   C. insulin
   B. glucagon   D. glucose

©2008 Pearson Education, Inc.
Anatomy & Physiology for Emergency Care, 2nd ed.

_____ 41. Another group of cells in the pancreas are called beta cells. They are responsible for producing _____.
A. glycogen
B. glucagon
C. insulin
D. glucose

_____ 42. Which of the following groups of cells require insulin or have insulin receptors present on the cell membrane?
A. neurons
B. red blood cells
C. skeletal muscle
D. epithelial cells in the kidney tubules

_____ 43. _____ is characterized by destruction of the beta cells of the pancreas.
A. Type I diabetes
B. Type II diabetes
C. Hypoglycemia
D. NIDDM

_____ 44. All of the following are risk factors for noninsulin-dependent diabetes (NIDDM) or Type II diabetes *except* _____.
A. family history
B. obesity
C. hypotension
D. hyperlipidemia

_____ 45. Which of the following diabetic conditions is also called insulin shock?
A. hyperglycemia
B. hypoglycemia
C. diabetic ketoacidosis
D. nonketonic hyperosmolar coma

_____ 46. Which of the following is released in response to a low level of oxygen in the kidneys?
A. calcitriol
B. erythropoietin
C. renin
D. angiotensin

_____ 47. _____ stimulates the release of aldosterone, which causes water and sodium retention.
A. Renin
B. Calcitriol
C. Angiotensin II
D. Erythropoietin

_____ 48. As you begin to eat a meal, _____ is released and it binds to neurons in the hypothalamus involved with emotion and appetite control. The result is a suppression of your appetite.
A. resistin
B. leptin
C. inhibin
D. insulin

_____ 49. The relationship between glucagon and insulin is an example of what type of pattern of hormonal interaction?
A. antagonistic effect
B. synergistic effect
C. permissive effect
D. integrative effect

_____ 50. Which of the following hormones plays a role in muscular and skeletal development?
A. growth hormone
B. insulin
C. parathyroid hormone
D. thyroid hormone

FILL IN THE BLANK

1. _____ cells are glandular cells that release their secretions directly into the extracellular fluid.

2. A _____ is a chemical messenger that is released in one tissue and transported by the blood to reach target cells in other tissues.

3. _____ activates kinase enzymes, which attach a high-energy phosphate group to another molecule in a process called phosphorylation.

4. The _____ is a slender stalk that connects the hypothalamus and the pituitary gland.

5. The hypothalamus secretes _____ that control the activity of endocrine cells.

6. The hypothalamus acts as an endocrine organ by synthesizing two hormones, _____ and _____.

7. The pituitary gland is a small oval gland that sets within a depression in the sphenoid bone called the _____.

8. _____ hormone targets the thyroid gland and triggers the release of thyroid hormones.

9. _____ hormone is responsible for sperm production in males.

10. _____ hormone stimulates cell growth and replication.

11. _____ are hormones that regulate the activities of male and female sex organs.

12. _____ hormone is important in the control of skin and hair pigmentation.

13. The other name for antidiuretic hormone (ADH) is _____.

14. _____ is a disease that occurs when the posterior pituitary gland no longer releases adequate amounts of ADH.

15. _____ cells are endocrine cells that produce the hormone calcitonin.

16. _____ disease occurs because of excessive release of thyroid hormone.

17. _____ crisis is a life-threatening endocrine emergency that can be fatal within 48 hours if untreated.

18. When calcium levels drop below normal, the chief cells of the thyroid gland release _____ to increase calcium levels in the body.

19. _____ is the principle mineralocortocoid found in the body.

20. Glucocorticoids affect glucose metabolism. The three most important glucocorticoids are _____, _____, and _____.

21. The adrenal medulla contains secretory cells that produce the two hormones _____ and _____.

22. The other term for Type I diabetes is _____.

23. _____ is a life-threatening condition that occurs from a deficiency of insulin.

24. _____ is released by specialized kidney cells in response to a decline in blood pressure or blood volume.

25. _____ stimulates the production of the mineralocortocoid aldosterone.

26. _____ is a hormone found in the heart that is released when excessive pressure occurs within the atria.

27. _____ is a hormone that reduces the body's sensitivity to insulin.

28. During stage I in the physiological response to stress, heart rate and blood pressure are elevated due to a release of _____ and _____.

29. The endocrine system undergoes few functional changes with age. The most dramatic is the decrease in the concentration of _____ hormones.

30. The two most common endocrine disorders in the elderly are _____ and _____.

MATCHING

Match the terms in Column A with the words or phrases in Column B. Write the letter of the corresponding words or phrases in the spaces provided.

Column A

_____ 1. adrenocorticotropic hormone

_____ 2. follicle-stimulating hormone

_____ 3. luteinizing hormone

_____ 4. prolactin

_____ 5. antidiuretic hormone

_____ 6. oxytocin

_____ 7. thyrotoxic crisis

_____ 8. myxedema coma

_____ 9. parathyroid hormone

_____ 10. aldosterone

Column B

a. released by posterior pituitary gland

b. stimulates smooth muscle contraction

c. caused by prolonged exposure to excessive thyroid hormones

d. stimulates the conservation of sodium

e. stimulates the production of milk

f. occurs from hypothyroidism

g. stimulates hormone release from adrenal cortex

h. stimulates kidneys to release calcitriol

i. promotes secretion of progesterone

j. stimulates secretion of estrogen

LABELING EXERCISE 10–1

Identify the parts of the endocrine system shown in Figure 10–1. Place the corresponding letter on the line next to the appropriate label.

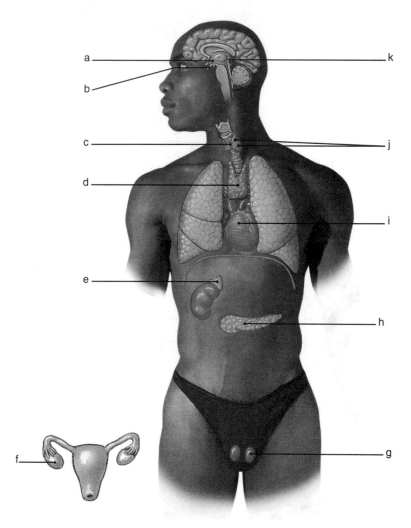

Figure 10–1 Endocrine System Overview

_____ 1. Thymus

_____ 2. Ovary

_____ 3. Hypothalamus

_____ 4. Heart

_____ 5. Pituitary gland

_____ 6. Pineal gland

_____ 7. Pancreatic islets

_____ 8. Parathyroid glands

_____ 9. Thyroid gland

_____ 10. Testis

_____ 11. Adrenal glands

LABELING EXERCISE 10–2

Part I

Using the illustration in Figure 10–2, identify the hormones released by the anterior and posterior pituitary glands. Place the corresponding letter on the line next to the appropriate label.

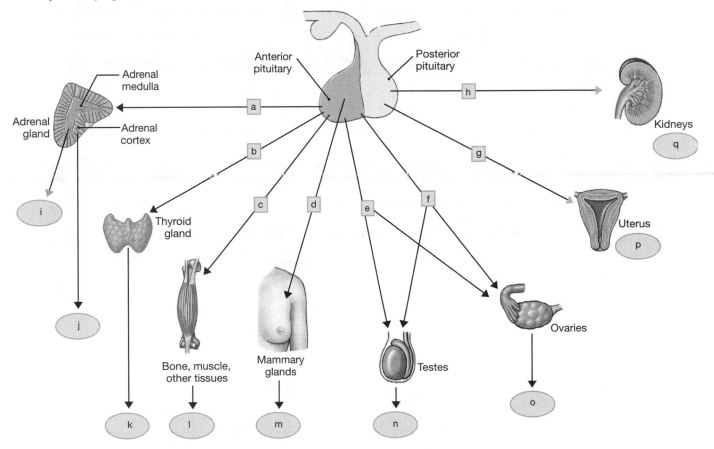

Figure 10–2 Hormones, Target Receptors and Actions

_____ 1. Antidiuretic hormone

_____ 2. Luteinizing hormone

_____ 3. Adrenocorticotropic hormone

_____ 4. Prolactin

_____ 5. Growth hormone

_____ 6. Thyroid-stimulating hormone

_____ 7. Oxytocin

_____ 8. Follicle-stimulating hormone

Part II

The pituitary hormones identified in Part I trigger the release of hormones from, or stimulate certain processes in, various organs in the body. Identify these using the illustration in Figure 10–2. Place the corresponding letter on the line next to the appropriate label.

_____ 1. Testosterone

_____ 2. Glucocorticoids (cortisol, corticosterone)

_____ 3. T_3, T_4

_____ 4. Epinephrine and norepinephrine

_____ 5. Progesterone

_____ 6. Milk production

_____ 7. Somatomedins

_____ 8. Contractions of smooth muscle

_____ 9. Water retention

SHORT ANSWER

1. You have a high school friend who calls you on the phone and tells you that he has been having problems with excessive thirst and frequent urination. Name the two disorders that could possibly cause this.

   _____

   _____

2. Describe in detail how a hormone binds to a cell membrane and triggers a second messenger inside the cell.

   _____

   _____

   _____

   _____

   _____

3. List the seven hormones released by the anterior pituitary gland and include the action of each.

   _____

   _____

   _____

   _____

   _____

   _____

   _____

   _____

4. List the two hormones produced by the posterior pituitary gland and include the action of each.

   _____

   _____

   _____

5. Discuss the differences between Cushing's syndrome and Addison's disease.

   _____

   _____

   _____

   _____

   _____

   _____

11 The Cardiovascular System: Blood

Chapter Objectives

1. Describe the important components and major functions of blood. — p. 408

2. Discuss the composition and functions of plasma. — pp. 408, 410

3. Describe the origins and production of the formed elements in blood. — pp. 410–411

4. Discuss the characteristics and functions of red blood cells. — pp. 411–412

5. Explain the factors that determine a person's blood type, and why blood types are important. — pp. 417–419

6. Categorize the various white blood cells on the basis of their structures and functions. — pp. 419–424

7. Describe the mechanisms that reduce blood loss after an injury. — pp. 425–428

Content Self-Evaluation

MULTIPLE CHOICE

_____ 1. Which of the following is *not* a function of blood?
   A. transport dissolved gases
   B. regulate pH
   C. restrict fluid loss through clotting
   D. All of the above are functions of blood.

_____ 2. _____ are *not* formed elements found in the blood.
   A. Platelets
   B. White blood cells
   C. Red blood cells
   D. Mast cells

_____ 3. Plasma comprises approximately what percentage of whole blood volume?
   A. 35 percent
   B. 45 percent
   C. 55 percent
   D. 65 percent

_____ 4. Plasma contains numerous proteins. Which of the following makes up roughly 60 percent of all plasma proteins?
   A. globulins
   B. antibodies
   C. albumins
   D. fibrinogen

_____ 5. Which of the following plasma proteins is responsible for blood clotting?
   A. globulins
   B. antibodies
   C. albumins
   D. fibrinogen

_____ 6. Which of the following plasma proteins is responsible for attacking pathogens?
A. globulins
B. antibodies
C. albumins
D. fibrinogen

_____ 7. The process by which formed elements are produced is called _____.
A. hemocytoblast
B. hemopoiesis
C. homeostasis
D. erythropoiesis

_____ 8. The percentage of whole blood made up of formed elements is called _____.
A. hemoglobin
B. hematocrit
C. hemocytoblast
D. hemopoiesis

_____ 9. The normal average hematocrit for an adult female is _____.
A. 40 percent
B. 42 percent
C. 46 percent
D. 50 percent

_____ 10. The _____ is (are) responsible for the red blood cell's ability to transport oxygen and carbon dioxide.
A. hemoglobin
B. leukocytes
C. platelets
D. hematocrit

_____ 11. Which of the following chemicals is essential for normal oxygen binding to the heme group of the hemoglobin?
A. copper
B. iron
C. zinc
D. nitrogen

_____ 12. The inherited disease sickle cell anemia occurs because of an abnormally shaped protein taking the place of one of the _____ chains.
A. alpha
B. beta
C. gamma
D. epsilon

_____ 13. The life span of a normal red blood cell is _____ days.
A. 90
B. 120
C. 150
D. 180

_____ 14. The life span of a sickled red blood cell is _____ days.
A. 5–10
B. 10–20
C. 30–40
D. 40–50

_____ 15. Patients who present with yellow or jaundiced skin do so because of a yellow-orange pigment called _____.
A. biliverdin
B. bilirubin
C. cyanosis
D. bile

_____ 16. At the end of the life span of a red blood cell, all of the following locations can break down the red blood cell _except_ the _____.
A. liver
B. spleen
C. bone marrow
D. pancreas

_____ 17. Erythropoiesis is the scientific term for the formation of _____.
A. white blood cells
B. platelets
C. red blood cells
D. mast cells

_____ 18. Erythropoietin is a hormone that is released from the _____ when oxygen concentrations decrease.
A. brain
B. liver
C. kidneys
D. bone marrow

_____ 19. Type A blood is blood that has _____.
A. A antibody
B. B antigen
C. A antigen
D. no antigen

_____ 20. Which type of blood is considered a universal donor?
   A. type O-negative   C. type B-negative
   B. type A-positive   D. type AB-positive

_____ 21. Which type of blood is considered a universal recipient?
   A. type O   C. type B
   B. type A   D. type AB

_____ 22. Which type of blood would be the best to give a patient suffering from a gunshot wound when the patient's blood type is unknown?
   A. type O   C. type B
   B. type A   D. type AB

_____ 23. The presence of the Rh factor on the red blood cell tells you whether or not you have the Rh _____.
   A. antigen   C. agglutinin
   B. antibody   D. pathogen

_____ 24. Which of the following is true regarding white blood cells or leukocytes?
   A. Leukocytes are smaller than red blood cells.
   B. Leukocytes contain hemoglobin.
   C. Leukocytes defend the body against pathogens.
   D. The most common leukocyte is the monocyte.

_____ 25. Which of the following white blood cells is _not_ capable of phagocytosis?
   A. lymphocytes   C. eosinophils
   B. neutrophils   D. monocytes

_____ 26. The most common white blood cell is the _____.
   A. lymphocyte   C. basophil
   B. neutrophil   D. monocyte

_____ 27. Which of the following white blood cells represents around 4 percent of the total white blood cells and increase during an allergic reaction?
   A. lymphocytes   C. eosinophils
   B. neutrophils   D. basophils

_____ 28. _____ are about twice the size of red blood cells and turn into a macrophage when they migrate out of the blood into the tissues.
   A. Lymphocytes   C. Monocytes
   B. Neutrophils   D. Eosinophils

_____ 29. _____ are the rarest of all white blood cells and release histamine during an inflammatory response.
   A. Lymphocytes   C. Basophils
   B. Monocytes   D. Eosinophils

_____ 30. _____ refers to an excessive amount of white blood cells and may indicate some form of leukemia.
   A. Leukopenia   C. Leukocytosis
   B. Lymphoiesis   D. Leukocyte

_____ 31. An abnormally low level of platelets is referred to as _____.
   A. thrombocytes   C. thrombocytosis
   B. megakaryocytes   D. thrombocytopenia

_____ 32. Which of the following is _not_ a phase of hemostasis?
   A. contraction of the smooth muscle of the blood vessel
   B. formation of a platelet plug
   C. release of thrombin to slow clotting cascade
   D. coagulation or blood clotting

_____ 33. The area of a blood vessel that is responsible for the majority of clotting can be found in the _____.
A. tunica media
B. tunica adventitia
C. epithelial layer
D. endothelial layer

_____ 34. Aspirin is a commonly used medicine given by paramedics to patients who may be suffering from an acute myocardial infarction. All of the following are effects of aspirin *except* _____.
A. inhibits platelet aggregation
B. antipyretic
C. blocks the formation of thromboxane A_2
D. increases the production of thromboxane A_2

_____ 35. Which of the following clotting pathways is the fastest?
A. common pathway
B. extrinsic pathway
C. intrinsic pathway
D. thrombin pathway

_____ 36. _____ is a protein and a precursor needed to form thrombin.
A. Fibrin
B. Fibrinogen
C. Prothrombin
D. Erythropoietin

_____ 37. _____ is an essential vitamin in almost every aspect of the clotting process.
A. Vitamin A
B. Vitamin B-12
C. Vitamin K
D. Vitamin C

_____ 38. _____ is a low-molecular weight form of heparin and is commonly used in the medical field.
A. Lovenox
B. Reopro
C. Plavix
D. Aggrastat

_____ 39. When a blood clot is no longer needed due to the repair process, the body releases a plasma protein called _____.
A. thrombin
B. fibrin
C. plasminogen
D. prothrombin

_____ 40. The activation of plasminogen produces an enzyme, which digests the fibrin strands of the clot. This enzyme is called _____.
A. prothrombin
B. thrombin
C. plasmin
D. fibrinogen

_____ 41. Blood clots that drift or move until they become stuck in a vessel are called _____.
A. thrombi
B. emboli
C. fibrin
D. plasmin

_____ 42. All of the following are examples of what can cause an emboli *except* _____.
A. air
B. fat
C. blood
D. All are examples.

_____ 43. Hemophilia is an inherited disorder characterized by an inadequate production of which clotting factor?
A. VI
B. VIII
C. IV
D. X

_____ 44. All of the following are diseases caused by an embolism *except* _____.
A. deep vein thrombosis
B. peripheral arterial occlusion
C. stroke
D. diabetes

_____ 45. All of the following are examples of fibrinolytic or thrombolytic drugs *except* _____.
A. tissue plasminogen activator
B. streptokinase
C. heparin
D. anistreplase

©2008 Pearson Education, Inc.
Anatomy & Physiology for Emergency Care, 2nd ed.

FILL IN THE BLANK

1. _____ contains dissolved proteins rather than a network of insoluble fibers.

2. _____ transport oxygen and carbon dioxide.

3. _____ function as part of the body's defense system.

4. _____ are the most abundant of all plasma proteins.

5. Streptokinase converts plasminogen to _____.

6. The _____ pathway begins with the activation of proenzymes exposed to collagen fibers at the injury site.

7. Embryonic blood cells travel to the liver, bone marrow, spleen, or thymus to become _____.

8. _____ are the most abundant blood cells.

9. _____ is an inherited disorder caused by abnormal hemoglobin.

10. Due to the lack of mitochondria, the red blood cell utilizes _____ as an energy source.

11. _____ is when red blood cells have a decreased hemoglobin content.

12. _____ are very immature red blood cells.

13. Erythropoietin has two major effects: _____ and _____.

14. The state of low tissue oxygen levels is called _____.

15. Type B blood has the _____ antigen present on the surface of the red blood cell.

16. If someone is given the wrong type of blood, a cross-reaction occurs which causes the blood to clump together. This is referred to as _____.

17. A macrophage is a _____ that has moved out of the bloodstream.

18. _____ are the largest of all white blood cells and are an aggressive phagocytic cell.

19. The process of lymphocyte production is called _____.

20. The other term for platelet is _____.

21. Platelets are manufactured in the bone marrow and remain in the circulation for an average of _____.

22. _____ is the process that halts or stops bleeding.

23. _____ converts the clotting protein prothrombin into the enzyme thrombin.

24. The two most frequently used medications for anticoagulation are _____ and _____.

25. The condition where a blood clot in the brain interrupts blood flow to a part of the brain is called a _____.

MATCHING

Match the terms in Column A with the words or phrases in Column B. Write the letter of the corresponding words or phrases in the spaces provided.

Column A

_____ 1. septicemia

_____ 2. phlebotomy

_____ 3. monocyte

_____ 4. hematuria

_____ 5. polycythemia

_____ 6. hemoglobin

_____ 7. basophil

_____ 8. leukopenia

_____ 9. calcium

_____ 10. pulmonary embolism

Column B

a. largest white blood cell

b. elevated hematocrit with normal blood volume

c. least common white blood cell

d. necessary for normal clotting

e. red blood cells present in urine

f. decrease in white blood cell production

g. withdraw blood from a vein

h. blood clot in the lung

i. bacterial toxins in the bloodstream

j. oxygen binding protein

LABELING EXERCISE 11–1

Identify the types of white blood cells shown in Figure 11–1. Place the corresponding letter on the line next to the appropriate label.

a

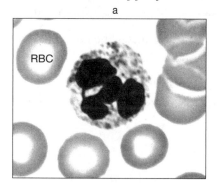

b

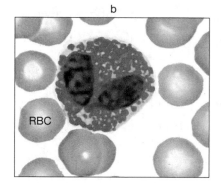

c

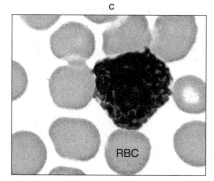

d

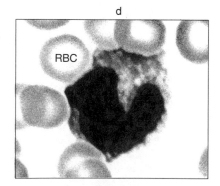

e

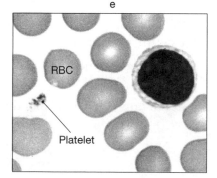

Figure 11–1 Types of White Blood Cells

_____ 1. Monocyte

_____ 2. Eosinophil

_____ 3. Neutrophil

_____ 4. Lymphocyte

_____ 5. Basophil

LABELING EXERCISE 11–2

Identify the events in the coagulation phase of hemostasis shown in Figure 11–2. Place the corresponding letter on the line next to the appropriate label. Please use each letter only once.

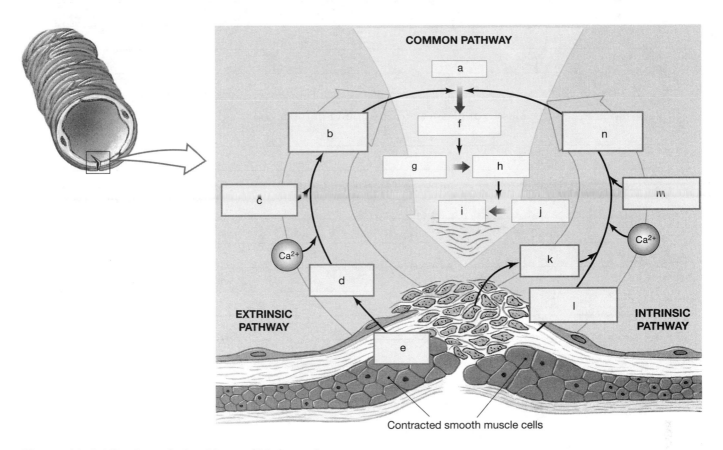

Figure 11–2 The Coagulation Phase of Hemostasis

_____ 1. Fibrin

_____ 2. Platelet factor

_____ 3. Multiple clotting factors

_____ 4. Thrombin

_____ 5. Prothrombin

_____ 6. Factor X

_____ 7. Prothrombinase

_____ 8. Tissue factors

_____ 9. Activated proenzymes

_____ 10. Fibrinogen

_____ 11. Factor X activator

_____ 12. Clotting factor VII

_____ 13. Tissue damage

_____ 14. Factor X activator

SHORT ANSWER

1. List the five primary functions of blood.

_____

_____

_____

_____

_____

2. What are the three classes of plasma proteins found in the blood?

_____

_____

3. List and describe all five of the different white blood cells.

_____

_____

_____

_____

_____

_____

_____

_____

_____

_____

_____

4. Compare and contrast the differences between red blood cells and white blood cells.

_____

_____

_____

_____

_____

5. Explain the role fibrinolytic, or thrombolytic, agents play in managing certain diseases.

_____

_____

_____

_____

_____

12 The Cardiovascular System: The Heart

Chapter Objectives

Content Self-Evaluation

MULTIPLE CHOICE

_____ 1. Which of the following chambers receives blood from the systemic circuit?
A. right atrium
B. left atrium
C. right ventricle
D. left ventricle

_____ 2. The heart is protected by a tough fibrous layer called the _____.
A. pericardium
B. myocardium
C. endocardium
D. epicardium

_____ 3. The inferior, pointed area of the heart is referred to as the _____.
A. base
B. apex
C. auricle
D. sulcus

_____ 4. The groove that marks the border between the atria and ventricles is called the _____.
A. apex
B. anterior interventricular sulcus
C. posterior interventricular sulcus
D. coronary sulcus

_____ 5. The innermost layer of the heart is called the _____.
   A. endocardium
   B. epicardium
   C. myocardium
   D. pericardium

_____ 6. The thickest of all muscle layers is called the _____.
   A. epicardium
   B. myocardium
   C. endocardium
   D. pericardium

_____ 7. The connective tissues of the heart provide all of the following *except* _____.
   A. provide support for cardiac muscle fibers
   B. add strength and prevent overexpansion
   C. increase oxygen availability to the heart
   D. help the heart return to normal shape after contraction

_____ 8. The _____ is a small hole that allows for blood to flow from the right atrium to the left atrium during embryonic development.
   A. fossa ovalis
   B. foramen ovale
   C. ductus arteriosus
   D. interatrial septum

_____ 9. The valve that is located between the right atrium and the right ventricle is called the _____ valve.
   A. mitral
   B. tricuspid
   C. bicuspid
   D. pulmonic

_____ 10. The valve that is located between the left atrium and left ventricle is called the _____ valve.
   A. aortic
   B. pulmonic
   C. mitral
   D. tricuspid

_____ 11. As blood is leaving the right ventricle, it must go through a valve on its way to the lungs. The name of the valve is the _____ valve.
   A. aortic
   B. pulmonary
   C. mitral
   D. bicuspid

_____ 12. The mitral and tricuspid valves rely on connective tissue fibers found within the ventricle that assist in the closing of the valve. These fibers are called _____.
   A. cusps
   B. papillary muscle
   C. chordae tendinae
   D. leaflets

_____ 13. The connective fibers that are attached to muscle extensions found within the ventricle are called _____ muscles.
   A. ventricular
   B. atrial
   C. papillary
   D. chordae

_____ 14. Certain valvular diseases impact the function of the valves. When chordae tendinae become loose or the valve does not completely close, there is some residual blood that flows back into the atrium. This is called _____.
   A. stenosis
   B. insufficiency
   C. regurgitation
   D. diastasis

_____ 15. The right and left coronary arteries originate at the base of the _____.
   A. pulmonary artery
   B. superior vena cava
   C. aorta
   D. inferior vena cava

_____ 16. The right coronary artery supplies blood to all of the following parts of the heart *except* the _____.
   A. right atrium
   B. right ventricle
   C. left ventricle
   D. It supplies blood to all of the above.

_____ 17. All of the following are risks factors for atherosclerosis *except* _____.
   A. age
   B. gender
   C. diabetes
   D. 2000 calorie-a-day diet

©2008 Pearson Education, Inc.
Anatomy & Physiology for Emergency Care, 2nd ed.

_____ 18. All of the following are symptoms that may be seen in a patient with acute coronary syndrome *except* _____.
A. chest pain
B. diaphoresis
C. nausea
D. abdominal pain

_____ 19. The use of a 12-lead ECG machine has become the standard when it comes to diagnosing a patient having an acute myocardial infarction. All of the following are changes on the ECG that would lead you to be suspicious of an acute myocardial infarction *except* _____.
A. ST elevation
B. new left bundle branch block
C. ST depression
D. All have the potential to be significant.

_____ 20. Glycoprotein IIb/IIIa inhibitors are relatively new drugs that have been shown to decrease platelet activity and response to a clot. An example of a glycoprotein IIb/IIIa inhibitor is _____.
A. aspirin
B. nitroglycerin
C. heparin
D. ReoPro

_____ 21. During depolarization, _____ enters the cell to change its membrane potential to positive.
A. calcium
B. sodium
C. potassium
D. chloride

_____ 22. During the plateau phase, _____ release causes the cardiac muscle to contract.
A. calcium
B. sodium
C. potassium
D. chloride

_____ 23. _____ leaves the cell during repolarization to restore the cell to a negative resting membrane potential.
A. Calcium
B. Sodium
C. Potassium
D. Chloride

_____ 24. Calcium is normally stored inside the cell within the _____.
A. nucleus
B. sarcoplasmic reticulum
C. mitochondria
D. Golgi apparatus

_____ 25. The complete depolarization-repolarization process in the cardiac muscle lasts _____ as long as the action potential in a skeletal muscle.
A. three times
B. 10 times
C. 20 times
D. 25 to 30 times

_____ 26. The primary pacemaker of the heart is considered the _____.
A. AV node
B. SA node
C. Purkinje fibers
D. AV bundle

_____ 27. The pacemaker cells within the SA node will normally fire _____ times a minute.
A. 70 to 80
B. 40 to 60
C. 20 to 40
D. 100 to 120

_____ 28. The pacemaker cells within the AV node normally fire _____ times a minute.
A. 60 to 100
B. 40 to 60
C. 70 to 80
D. 20 to 40

_____ 29. The amount of time it takes a stimulus to travel from the SA node to the AV node is roughly _____.
A. 40 msec.
B. 50 msec.
C. 60 msec.
D. 70 msec.

_____ 30. _____ is a condition in which the heart rate is slower than normal.
A. Tachycardia
B. Ectopic
C. Bradycardia
D. Tachypnea

_____ 31. Depolarization of the atria is represented on the ECG as a _____.
   A. T wave
   B. P wave
   C. QRS complex
   D. S wave

_____ 32. Depolarization of the ventricles is represented on the ECG as a _____.
   A. T wave
   B. P wave
   C. QRS complex
   D. U wave

_____ 33. Repolarization of the ventricles is represented on the ECG as a _____.
   A. T wave
   B. P wave
   C. QRS Complex
   D. S wave

_____ 34. The term used to describe contraction of the cardiac muscle is _____.
   A. diastole
   B. asystole
   C. systole
   D. diastasis

_____ 35. The term used to describe relaxation of the cardiac muscle is _____.
   A. diastole
   B. asystole
   C. systole
   D. cardiac cycle

_____ 36. During systole, which of the following heart valves is open?
   A. mitral
   B. tricuspid
   C. aortic
   D. bicuspid

_____ 37. During diastole, which of the following valves are open?
   A. mitral
   B. pulmonary
   C. aortic
   D. systemic

_____ 38. Which of the following parts of the cardiac cycle occur during atrial systole?
   A. semilunar valves open
   B. ventricles completely fill with blood
   C. mitral and tricuspid valve close
   D. ventricles relax

_____ 39. Which of the following parts of the cardiac cycle occur during ventricular systole?
   A. ventricles completely fill with blood
   B. pulmonary and aortic valves close
   C. mitral and tricuspid valves open
   D. pulmonary and aortic valves open

_____ 40. Which of the following equations is true regarding cardiac output?
   A. $CO = PVR \times HR$
   B. $CO = PVR \times SV$
   C. $CO = SV \times HR$
   D. $CO = EF \times HR$

_____ 41. The amount of blood ejected from the heart during a single contraction is called the
   _____.
   A. cardiac output
   B. blood pressure
   C. stroke volume
   D. heart rate

_____ 42. The correct order through the cardiac conducting system is _____.
   A. SA node, AV node, Purkinje fibers, right and left bundle branches
   B. AV node, SA node, bundle of His, Purkinje fibers, right and left bundle branches
   C. SA node, AV node, bundle of His, right and left bundle branches, Purkinje fibers
   D. AV node, SA node, bundle of His, right and left bundle branches, Purkinje fibers

_____ 43. The _____ reflex produces adjustments in the heart rate based on venous return.
   A. cardiac
   B. ventricular
   C. Bainbridge
   D. venous

_____ 44. The _____ principle states that the more you stretch the cardiac muscle, the greater
   the force of contraction.
   A. Bainbridge
   B. Starks
   C. Frank-Starling
   D. stroke volume

_____ 45. The release of acetylcholine from the parasympathetic nervous system will have what effect on the heart rate?
A. speed the rate up
B. no effect at all
C. slow the rate down
D. Aacetylcholine only impacts contraction, not rate.

_____ 46. The release of epinephrine from the sympathetic nervous system will have what effect on the heart rate?
A. speed the rate up
B. no effect at all
C. slow the rate down
D. Eepinephrine affects only the speed of conduction, not rate.

_____ 47. What part of the brain has receptors that help regulate the rate of the heart?
A. cerebrum
B. cerebellum
C. medulla
D. thalamus

_____ 48. Digitalis is a medication that works by increasing the amount of _____ in the cardiac muscle, which leads to a stronger force of contraction.
A. calcium
B. sodium
C. potassium
D. magnesium

_____ 49. Which of the following electrolyte imbalances can cause cardiac muscle contraction to be weak and irregular?
A. hypocalcemia
B. hypercalcemia
C. hypokalemia
D. hyperkalemia

_____ 50. As the core temperature of the body decreases, all of the following commonly occur except _____.
A. SA node rate slows down
B. heart rate slows down
C. force of contraction decreases
D. force of contraction increases

ORDERING EXERCISE

Place the following steps of the normal cardiac cycle in the correct order using the letters A–E.

_____ 1. As pressure in the ventricles rise above the pressure in the atria, the AV valves close.

_____ 2. Ventricular diastole begins as the ventricular pressure begins to drop and the semilunar valves close.

_____ 3. The ventricles are partially filled with blood. The atria contract and push the remaining blood into the ventricles.

_____ 4. The increased pressure in the ventricles forces the semilunar valves open and blood flows through the pulmonic and aortic valves. This continues throughout ventricular systole.

_____ 5. Ventricular pressures begin to drop. As the pressure drops below atrial pressures, the AV valves open up and blood flows from the atria to the ventricles.

FILL IN THE BLANK

1. _____ carry blood away from the heart.

2. _____ are thin-walled vessels found between the smallest arteries and smallest veins.

3. A fibrous sac called the _____ protects the heart.

4. The _____ and _____ mark the boundary between the right and left ventricles.

5. The _____ is the outermost muscle layer of the heart.

6. The _____ is the innermost muscular layer of the heart.

7. _____ are interlocking membranes that act like gap junctions and allow for an organized contraction of the heart.

8. The large veins that bring blood back to the right part of the heart are called the _____.

9. The _____ allows blood to travel from the right atrium to the left atrium while the lungs are developing prior to birth.

10. _____ is the chest pain that results from temporary ischemia to the heart during stress.

11. The _____ valve is found between the left ventricle and the systemic circulation.

12. One of the most common valve disorders is mitral valve prolapse. It is most commonly caused by _____ or _____.

13. The right and left coronary arteries originate at the _____.

14. The _____ artery has the marginal and the posterior descending artery as branches.

15. The _____ artery has the circumflex and anterior descending artery as branches.

16. When a part of the heart dies from a lack of blood supply, this is called a _____.

17. The progressive buildup of fatty streaks and endothelial injury to an artery is called _____.

18. Two common dysrhythmias associated with myocardial ischemia and death are _____ and _____.

19. The two most significant findings on the 12-lead ECG that would lead you to believe that a patient has had an acute myocardial infarction are _____ or _____.

20. _____ involves inserting a small catheter into an affected coronary artery.

21. _____ rushes into the cardiac muscle cell during depolarization.

22. _____ is a faster than normal heart rate.

23. Patients who are at risk for sudden cardiac death have an _____ implanted in case the patient has a life-threatening dysrhythmia.

24. The amount of blood pumped by each ventricle in one minute is called the _____.

25. The amount of blood ejected from the ventricles in a single beat is called the _____.

26. A myocardial concussion or _____ occurs when there is a blow to the myocardium but no noticeable injury can be found.

27. The _____ states that the more the myocardium is stretched, the better the force of the contraction.

28. _____ is a disorder caused by abnormal functioning of one of the cardiac valves.

29. _____ is a major procedure that requires that the sternum be split, the heart stopped (cardioplegia), and the patient placed on a bypass pump for the duration of the surgery.

30. Higher than normal potassium levels or _____ could lead to life-threatening dysrhythmias.

©2008 Pearson Education, Inc.
Anatomy & Physiology for Emergency Care, 2nd ed.

MATCHING

Match the terms in Column A with the words or phrases in Column B. Write the letter of the corresponding words or phrases in the spaces provided.

Column A

_____ 1. pericardium

_____ 2. myocardium

_____ 3. defibrillator

_____ 4. defibrillation

_____ 5. cardiac arrhythmia

_____ 6. pericarditis

_____ 7. prolapse

_____ 8. cardiac tamponade

_____ 9. ST elevation

_____ 10. intercalated discs

Column B

a. device used to eliminate ventricular fibrillation

b. inflammation of the pericardium

c. valve does not close properly

d. lines the pericardial cavity

e. fluid accumulation in pericardial sac

f. thick middle layer of muscle

g. treatment for ventricular fibrillation

h. seen on EKG during an MI

i. only found in cardiac muscle

j. abnormal pattern of cardiac electrical activity

LABELING EXERCISE 12–1

Identify the heart's major anterior surface features shown in Figure 12–1. Place the corresponding letter on the line next to the appropriate label.

_____ 1. Fat in anterior interventricular sulcus

_____ 2. Superior vena cava

_____ 3. Pulmonary trunk

_____ 4. Aorta

_____ 5. Left pulmonary artery

_____ 6. Fat in coronary sulcus

_____ 7. Auricle of left atrium

_____ 8. Auricle of right atrium

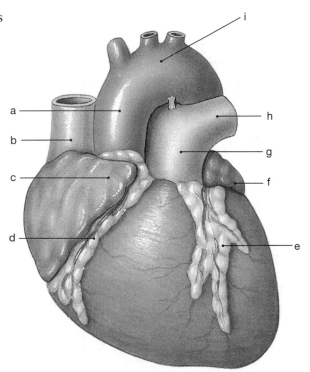

Figure 12–1 Surface Anatomy of the Heart–Anterior View

LABELING EXERCISE 12–2

Identify the heart's major posterior surface features shown in Figure 12–2. Place the corresponding letter on the line next to the appropriate label.

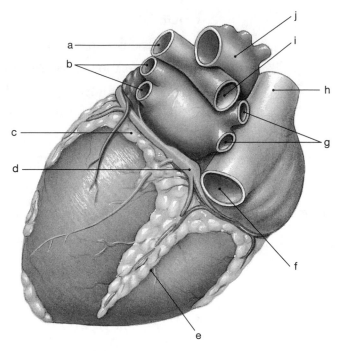

Figure 12–2 Surface Anatomy of the Heart–Posterior View

_____ 1. Right pulmonary veins

_____ 2. Right pulmonary artery

_____ 3. Inferior vena cava

_____ 4. Fat in coronary sulcus

_____ 5. Left pulmonary veins

_____ 6. Arch of aorta

_____ 7. Superior vena cava

_____ 8. Left pulmonary artery

_____ 9. Coronary sinus

_____ 10. Fat in posterior interventricular sulcus

LABELING EXERCISE 12-3

Identify the heart's major internal landmarks shown in Figure 12–3. Place the corresponding letter on the line next to the appropriate label.

_____ 1. Papillary muscles

_____ 2. Cusp of right AV (tricuspid) valve

_____ 3. Interventricular septum

_____ 4. Cusp of the left AV (bicuspid) valve

_____ 5. Opening of the coronary sinus

_____ 6. Interatrial septum

_____ 7. Right ventricle

_____ 8. Left pulmonary arteries

_____ 9. Fossa ovalis

_____ 10. Left ventricle

_____ 11. Pulmonary trunk

_____ 12. Superior vena cava

_____ 13. Aortic arch

_____ 14. Inferior vena cava

_____ 15. Pulmonary semilunar valve

_____ 16. Right pulmonary arteries

_____ 17. Left pulmonary veins

_____ 18. Aorta

_____ 19. Aortic semilunar valve

_____ 20. Right atrium

_____ 21. Chordae tendinae

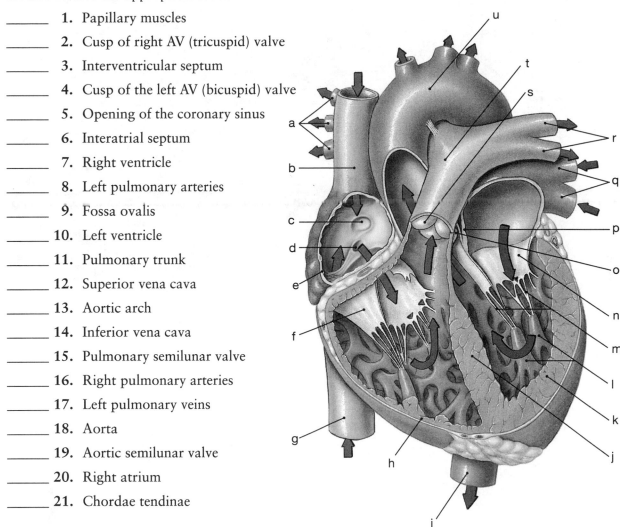

Figure 12–3 Sectional Anatomy of the Heart

LABELING EXERCISE 12–4

Identify the heart valves shown in Figure 12–4. Place the corresponding letter on the line next to the appropriate label.

_____ 1. Pulmonary semilunar valve-closed

_____ 2. Left AV (bicuspid) valve-closed

_____ 3. Left AV (bicuspid) valve-open

_____ 4. Aortic semilunar valve-open

_____ 5. Aortic semilunar valve-closed

_____ 6. Pulmonary semilunar valve-open

_____ 7. Right AV (tricuspid) valve-open

_____ 8. Right AV (tricuspid) valve-closed

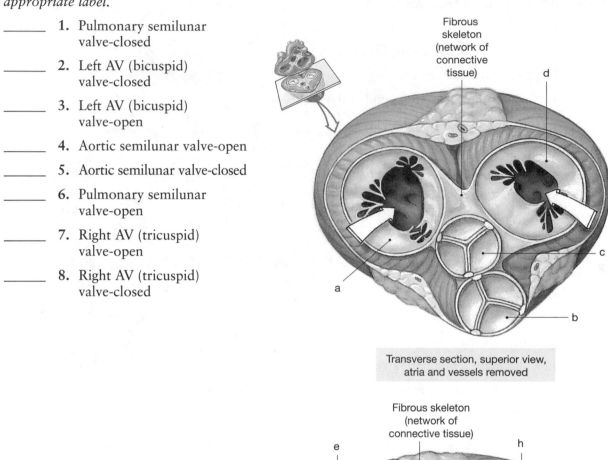

Transverse section, superior view, atria and vessels removed

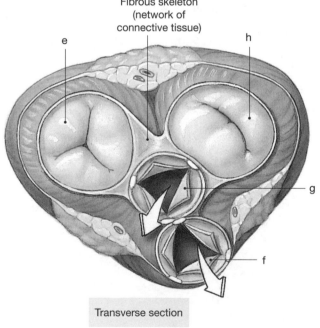

Transverse section

Figure 12–4 Valves of the Heart

LABELING EXERCISE 12–5

Identify the blood vessels that constitute the coronary circulation (anterior view) shown in Figure 12–5. Place the corresponding letter on the line next to the appropriate label.

_____ 1. Anterior interventricular branch of left coronary artery (LCA)

_____ 2. Marginal branch of the right coronary artery (RCA)

_____ 3. Left coronary artery

_____ 4. Anterior cardiac veins

_____ 5. Pulmonary trunk

_____ 6. Left atrium

_____ 7. Aorta

_____ 8. Small cardiac vein

_____ 9. Circumflex branch of left coronary artery (LCA)

_____ 10. Right coronary artery (RCA)

_____ 11. Great cardiac vein

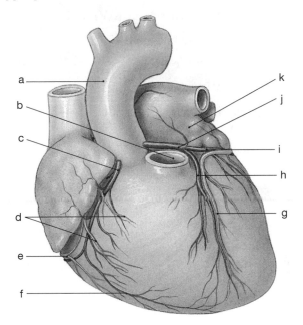

Figure 12–5 Coronary Circulation–Anterior View

LABELING EXERCISE 12–6

Identify the blood vessels that constitute the coronary circulation (posterior view) shown in Figure 12–6. Place the corresponding letter on the line next to the appropriate label.

_____ 1. Marginal branch of right coronary artery (RCA)

_____ 2. Great cardiac vein

_____ 3. Right coronary artery (RCA)

_____ 4. Posterior cardiac vein

_____ 5. Small cardiac vein

_____ 6. Posterior left ventricular branch of the left coronary artery (LCA)

_____ 7. Coronary sinus

_____ 8. Posterior interventricular branch of right coronary artery (RCA)

_____ 9. Circumflex branch of left coronary artery (LCA)

_____ 10. Middle cardiac vein

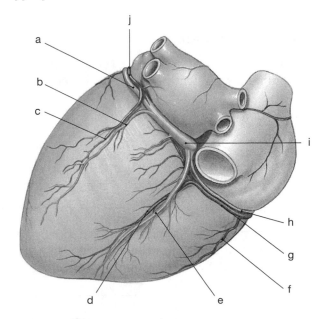

Figure 12–6 Coronary Circulation–Posterior View

LABELING EXERCISE 12–7

Identify the elements of the conducting system shown in Figure 12–7. Place the corresponding letter on the line next to the appropriate label.

_____ 1. Atrioventricular (AV) node

_____ 2. Bundle branches

_____ 3. Purkinje fibers

_____ 4. AV bundle

_____ 5. Sinoatrial (SA) node

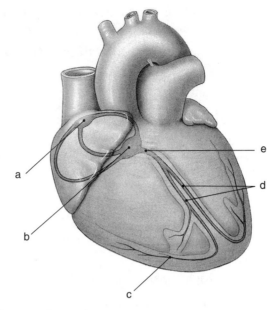

Figure 12–7 The Conducting System of the Heart

SHORT ANSWER

1. Starting at the right atrium, trace the flow of a drop of blood through the heart and pulmonary/systemic systems back to the right atrium. Include all of the valves.

   _____

   _____

   _____

   _____

   _____

   _____

2. Starting at the SA node, name all of the parts of the electrical conduction system of the heart in the order the electricity normally travels.

   _____

   _____

   _____

   _____

   _____

3. List the signs and symptoms a patient may experience who has an acute coronary syndrome. Also discuss the common complications seen.

_____

_____

_____

_____

_____

4. Discuss the three phases of the action potential of the cardiac muscle cell.

_____

_____

_____

_____

_____

_____

5. Describe the role of the sympathetic and parasympathetic nervous systems on the heart.

_____

_____

_____

_____

_____

13 The Cardiovascular System: Blood Vessels and Circulation

Chapter Objectives

Content Self-Evaluation

MULTIPLE CHOICE

_____ 1. Which of the following represent the flow of blood in the microcirculatory network?
A. veins → venules → capillaries → arterioles → arteries
B. arteries → arterioles → capillaries → venules → veins
C. capillaries → venules → veins → arterioles → arteries
D. capillaries → arterioles → arteries → venules → veins

_____ 2. The innermost layer of an artery is called the _____.
A. tunica intima
B. tunica media
C. tunica externa
D. tunica adventitia

_____ 3. The middle layer of a vessel, which contains most of the smooth muscle, is called the _____.
A. tunica intima
B. tunica media
C. tunica externa
D. tunica adventitia

_____ 4. Blood vessels that have a valve to prevent backflow are called _____.
A. arteries
B. veins
C. capillaries
D. arterioles

_____ 5. The blood vessels that have the biggest impact on blood pressure are the _____.
A. arteries
B. veins
C. venules
D. capillaries

_____ 6. The vessels that carry blood back to the heart are called _____.
A. arteries
B. veins
C. capillaries
D. arterioles

_____ 7. The process where the arterial walls become thick and less elastic is called _____.
A. atherosclerosis
B. calcification
C. arteriosclerosis
D. inflammation

_____ 8. All of the following increase the development of atherosclerosis _except_ _____.
A. diabetes
B. hypotension
C. stress
D. smoking

_____ 9. The entrance into each capillary is guarded by a band of smooth muscle that reduces the flow of blood into the capillary. This is called the _____.
A. capillary bed
B. postcapillary sphincter
C. precapillary sphincter
D. vasomotor sphincter

_____ 10. The difference between the systolic pressure and the diastolic pressure is called the _____.
A. pulsus alternans
B. pulsus paradoxsus
C. pulse pressure
D. blood pressure

_____ 11. You are caring for a patient complaining of chest pain. The patient's blood pressure is 126/78. What is the patient's pulse pressure?
A. 48
B. 204
C. 1.6
D. 24

_____ 12. By the time blood reaches the precapillary sphincter, the pressure in the vessels has _____.
A. stayed roughly the same
B. increased
C. dropped slightly
D. decreased significantly

©2008 Pearson Education, Inc.
Anatomy & Physiology for Emergency Care, 2nd ed.

_____ 13. Which of the following blood pressures would you consider to be hypertensive?
   A. 110/80   C. 140/90
   B. 100/66   D. 138/76

_____ 14. Continuous movement and exchange of water and solutes helps the capillaries to maintain homeostasis. This important exchange does all of the following *except* _____.
   A. maintain communication between plasma and interstitial fluid
   B. speed the distribution of nutrients to the cells
   C. assist in the movement of soluble proteins that cannot cross capillary walls
   D. flush out bacterial toxins

_____ 15. The movement of materials across the capillary wall occurs by all of the following methods *except* _____.
   A. osmosis   C. active transport
   B. diffusion   D. filtration

_____ 16. Capillary hydrostatic pressure moves water _____.
   A. into the capillary   C. into the blood
   B. out of the capillary   D. into the interstitial fluid

_____ 17. Blood osmotic pressure tends to _____.
   A. reabsorb water back into the blood   C. push fluid into the capillary
   B. reabsorb solutes from the fluid   D. push solutes into the capillary

_____ 18. The average pressure found within the right atrium is _____.
   A. 2 mm/Hg   C. 6 mm/Hg
   B. 4 mm/Hg   D. 8 mm/Hg

_____ 19. When assessing a patient's blood pressure, you will normally hear Korotkoff sounds during the process. What are Korotkoff sounds?
   A. the first sound heard or the systolic pressure
   B. the sound heard when above 200 mm/Hg
   C. the sound heard as the pressure in the cuff falls below the systolic pressure
   D. the sound heard as the pressure in the cuff falls below the diastolic pressure

_____ 20. The mechanisms involved in the regulation of cardiovascular functions include _____.
   A. cardiac output and heart rate
   B. peripheral resistance
   C. autoregulation, neural mechanisms, and endocrine mechanisms
   D. respirations and heart rate

_____ 21. High shear forces within the capillaries or the presence of histamine during inflammation triggers the release of the important vasodilating agent _____.
   A. dopamine   C. nitric oxide
   B. serotonin   D. oxygen

_____ 22. The vasomotor centers found within the medulla oblongata of the brain primarily control _____.
   A. the diameter of the venules through sympathetic innervation
   B. the diameter of the arterioles through parasympathetic innervation
   C. the diameter of the arterioles through sympathetic innervation
   D. the diameter of the venules through parasympathetic innervation

_____ 23. The baroreceptors in the heart are located in the _____.
   A. vena cava, carotid sinus, and left atrium
   B. vena cava, carotid sinus, and right atrium
   C. aortic sinuses, carotid sinuses, and right atrium
   D. aortic sinus, vena cava, and right atrium

_____ 24. If blood pressure falls below normal, all of the following occur *except* _____.
   A. increase in cardiac output
   B. vasoconstriction
   C. increase in SA node activity
   D. decrease in stroke volume

_____ 25. Chemoreceptors found within the carotid and aortic bodies respond to carbon dioxide, oxygen, and pH levels in the _____.
   A. blood
   B. cerebrospinal fluid
   C. interstitial fluid
   D. both A and B

_____ 26. Antidiuretic hormone (ADH) is released from the posterior pituitary gland for all of the following reasons *except* _____.
   A. decrease in blood volume
   B. increase in the osmotic concentration of the plasma
   C. presence of angiotensin II
   D. presence of angiotensin I

_____ 27. All of the following will cause an increase in blood pressure *except* an _____.
   A. increase in aldosterone
   B. increase in atrial natriuretic peptide
   C. increase in angiotensin II
   D. increase in blood volume

_____ 28. Which of the following hormones stimulates thirst?
   A. renin
   B. aldosterone
   C. angiotensin I
   D. angiotensinogen

_____ 29. Atrial natriuretic peptide is a hormone that does all of the following *except* _____.
   A. promotes water loss through the kidneys
   B. stimulates the release of ADH
   C. blocks aldosterone release
   D. reduces thirst

_____ 30. During exercise, both the cardiac output and blood distribution patterns change. During exercise, which of the following are changes that are typically seen?
   A. Capillary blood flow increases.
   B. Venous return to the heart increases.
   C. Breathing rate increases.
   D. All of the above occur.

_____ 31. Blood pressure will elevate with an increase in _____.
   A. cardiac output
   B. peripheral vascular resistance
   C. blood volume
   D. All of the above are correct.

_____ 32. In the case of significant blood loss, all of the following are normal responses *except* _____.
   A. sympathetic nervous system releases epinephrine and norepinephrine
   B. kidney releases renin to increase angiotensin II activity
   C. ADH is released from the posterior pituitary gland
   D. parasympathetic nervous system releases acetylcholine to increase heart rate

_____ 33. Which of the following types of shock is caused by a loss of autonomic control of the peripheral blood vessels?
   A. hypovolemic
   B. anaphylactic
   C. neurogenic
   D. septic

_____ 34. Which of the following types of shock is caused by a release of histamine into the circulation?
   A. hypovolemic
   B. anaphylactic
   C. neurogenic
   D. septic

_____ 35. All of the following are signs and symptoms of shock *except* _____.
   A. pale, cool skin
   B. weak, rapid pulse
   C. increase in urination
   D. fall in blood pressure

_____ 36. The only artery that carries unoxygenated blood is the _____.
A. cerebral artery
B. pulmonary artery
C. brachial artery
D. subclavian artery

_____ 37. A 40-year-old patient has been involved in an auto accident with significant damage to the car. When you arrive at the hospital, the doctor tells you that it looks like the patient has an aneurysm. What type of aneurysm do you think this patient has?
A. atherosclerotic
B. infectious
C. dissecting
D. traumatic

_____ 38. All of the following are signs or symptoms of an abdominal aneurysm _except_

_____.
A. chest pain
B. hypotension
C. back pain
D. urge to defecate

_____ 39. Which group of arteries originates off of the aortic arch?
A. right carotid, right subclavian, and anterior communicating artery
B. right carotid, right brachial, and right subclavian
C. brachiocephalic trunk, left carotid, and left subclavian
D. brachiocephalic trunk, right carotid, and right subclavian

_____ 40. The subclavian artery immediately branches into the _____.
A. brachial artery
B. radial artery
C. ulnar artery
D. axillary artery

_____ 41. The basilar and internal carotid arteries form an interconnected circle of blood supply to the brain to reduce the likelihood of circulatory impairment. This structure is called the _____.
A. basilar artery structure
B. internal carotid artery structure
C. circle of Willis
D. circle of Dupont

_____ 42. All of the following arteries are responsible for providing blood to the digestive organs _except_ the _____.
A. celiac artery
B. superior mesenteric artery
C. inferior mesenteric artery
D. phrenic artery

_____ 43. The _____ arteries originate between the superior and inferior mesenteric arteries.
A. suprarenal
B. gonadal
C. iliac
D. lumbar

_____ 44. When the femoral artery reaches the back of the knee, it becomes the _____ artery.
A. anterior tibial
B. posterior tibial
C. popliteal
D. fibular

_____ 45. One of the most easily accessible veins in the arm to start an IV can be found between the brachial and basilic veins. It is called the _____.
A. radial vein
B. axillary vein
C. brachial vein
D. median cubital vein

_____ 46. The superior vena cava receives blood from the thoracic cage from the _____.
A. subclavian vein
B. azygos vein
C. brachial vein
D. axillary vein

_____ 47. In fetal circulation, there is an opening between the pulmonary artery and the aorta to allow for oxygenated blood to come from the mother to the baby. The hole is called the

_____.
A. fossa ovalis
B. foramen magnum
C. ductus arteriosus
D. ligamentum arteriosum

_____ 48. The umbilical cord contains _____.
   A. one artery and one vein
   B. two veins and one artery
   C. two arteries and one vein
   D. two arteries and two veins

_____ 49. Age-related circulation issues include all of the following *except* _____.
   A. decrease in hematocrit
   B. pooling of blood in distal veins
   C. constriction of veins by a small thrombus
   D. increase in hemoglobin concentration

_____ 50. In the heart, the age related changes include all of the following *except* _____.
   A. a reduction in cardiac output
   B. replacement of damaged cardiac muscle with functional muscle
   C. progressive atherosclerosis
   D. changes in nodal activity

FILL IN THE BLANK

1. Blood flowing out of the capillary network first enters the _____.

2. A _____ is a device that is used to measure blood pressure.

3. _____ is an abnormal accumulation of fluid in peripheral tissues.

4. _____ is a progressive disease with thickening of the vessel wall.

5. Sometimes blood vessels provide an alternate route for blood to flow by forming an _____.

6. Veins utilize _____ to help overcome the force of gravity on blood flow.

7. The resistance of the arterial system is called _____.

8. _____ is the resistance to flow that results from interactions among molecules and suspended materials in a liquid.

9. _____ is a condition in which the hematocrit is reduced due to inadequate production of hemoglobin.

10. Systemic pressures are the highest in the aorta at around _____ mm/Hg and the lowest at the vena cavae at about _____ mm/Hg.

11. By the time blood reaches the _____, the pressure has fallen to 35 mm/Hg.

12. A consistent elevation in blood pressure is called _____.

13. Blood pressure is a function of _____ and _____.

14. Three variables influence blood flow: _____, _____ and _____.

15. Chemicals or factors that dilate the precapillary sphincter are called _____.

16. The baroreceptors involved in cardiovascular regulation are located in the _____ and _____ sinuses.

17. The hormones that are released for short-term cardiovascular regulation are _____ and _____.

18. _____ is released from the posterior pituitary gland in response to a decrease in blood volume.

19. _____ is formed in the blood following the release of renin.

20. Erythropoietin is released by the _____ when the blood pressure falls or oxygen content in the blood becomes abnormally low.

21. _____ is produced by specialized cells in the atrial walls when blood pressure increases.

22. _____ is a state of inadequate tissue perfusion.

23. _____ occurs when a blood clot or other particle lodges in the pulmonary artery.

24. Blood coming back to the heart from the lungs travels through the _____ before entering the left atria.

25. An _____ is a bulging in the weakened wall of a blood vessel.

26. The brachiocephalic trunk ascends for a short distance before turning into the _____ and _____.

27. The brachial artery branches to create the _____ and _____ arteries.

28. The _____ is a ring shaped arterial structure that encircles the stalk of the pituitary gland.

29. The _____ arteries deliver blood to the diaphragm.

30. _____ is a type of vasculitis that is characterized by episodes of pain and cyanosis in the fingers and toes.

31. In fetal circulation, some of the blood flows through the capillaries, but the rest reaches the inferior vena cava through the _____.

32. Prior to birth, the small elongated hole found between the right and left atria is called the _____.

33. The small fetal connection between the pulmonary artery and the aorta is called the _____.

34. The elderly are at risk for _____ because of their sedentary lifestyle.

35. An aortic rupture or tear from trauma has a _____ percentage mortality rate.

MATCHING

Match the terms in Column A with the words or phrases in Column B. Write the letter of the corresponding words or phrases in the spaces provided.

Column A

_____ 1. plaque

_____ 2. anastomosis

_____ 3. vasculitis

_____ 4. renin

_____ 5. circle of Willis

_____ 6. axillary artery

_____ 7. iliac artery

_____ 8. popliteal artery

_____ 9. Homan's sign

_____ 10. phlebitis

Column B

a. inflammation of a blood vessel

b. provides blood to pelvis

c. precursor to angiotensin

d. branch after femoral artery

e. test for deep vein thrombosis

f. inflammation of vein

g. fatty mass of tissue that occludes lumen of vessel

h. encircles the pituitary gland

i. the joining of two vessels or tubes

j. branch before brachial artery

LABELING EXERCISE 13–1

Identify the parts of the arterial system shown in Figure 13–1. Place the corresponding letter on the line next to the appropriate label.

_____ 1. Plantar arch

_____ 2. Brachiocephalic trunk

_____ 3. Femoral

_____ 4. Anterior tibial

_____ 5. Celiac trunk

_____ 6. Internal iliac

_____ 7. Inferior mesenteric

_____ 8. Ascending aorta

_____ 9. Superior mesenteric

_____ 10. Descending aorta

_____ 11. Palmar arches

_____ 12. Left subclavian

_____ 13. Aortic arch

_____ 14. Vertebral

_____ 15. Popliteal

_____ 16. Gonadal

_____ 17. Right common carotid

_____ 18. Left common carotid

_____ 19. Posterior tibial

_____ 20. Axillary

_____ 21. Brachial

_____ 22. Ulnar

_____ 23. Renal

_____ 24. External iliac

_____ 25. Common iliac

_____ 26. Deep femoral

_____ 27. Right subclavian

_____ 28. Dorsalis pedis

_____ 29. Fibular

_____ 30. Radial

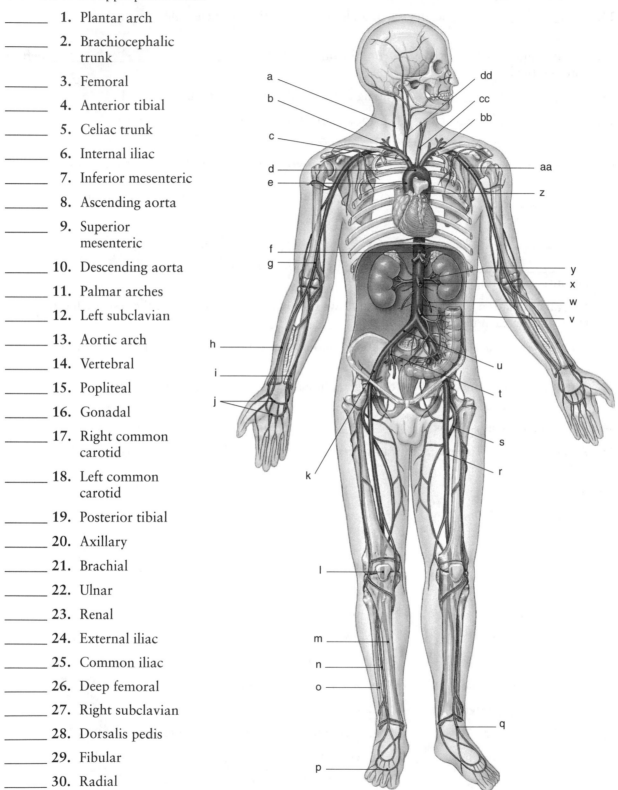

Figure 13–1 An Overview of the Arterial System

©2008 Pearson Education, Inc.
Anatomy & Physiology for Emergency Care, 2nd ed.

LABELING EXERCISE 13–2

Identify the parts of the venous system shown in Figure 13–2. Place the corresponding letter on the line next to the appropriate label.

_____ 1. Fibular

_____ 2. Digital veins

_____ 3. Basilic

_____ 4. Internal iliac

_____ 5. Cephalic

_____ 6. Lumbar

_____ 7. Renal

_____ 8. Popliteal

_____ 9. Axillary

_____ 10. Median cubital

_____ 11. Subclavian

_____ 12. Femoral

_____ 13. Intercostals

_____ 14. Palmar venous arches

_____ 15. Posterior tibial

_____ 16. Brachiocephalic

_____ 17. External jugular

_____ 18. External iliac

_____ 19. Median antebrachial

_____ 20. Great saphenous

_____ 21. Plantar venous arch

_____ 22. Vertebral

_____ 23. Internal jugular

_____ 24. Ulnar

_____ 25. Inferior vena cava

_____ 26. Superior vena cava

_____ 27. Brachial

_____ 28. Radial

_____ 29. Small saphenous

_____ 30. Left and right common iliac

_____ 31. Anterior tibial

_____ 32. Deep femoral

_____ 33. Hepatics

_____ 34. Gonadal

_____ 35. Dorsal venous arch

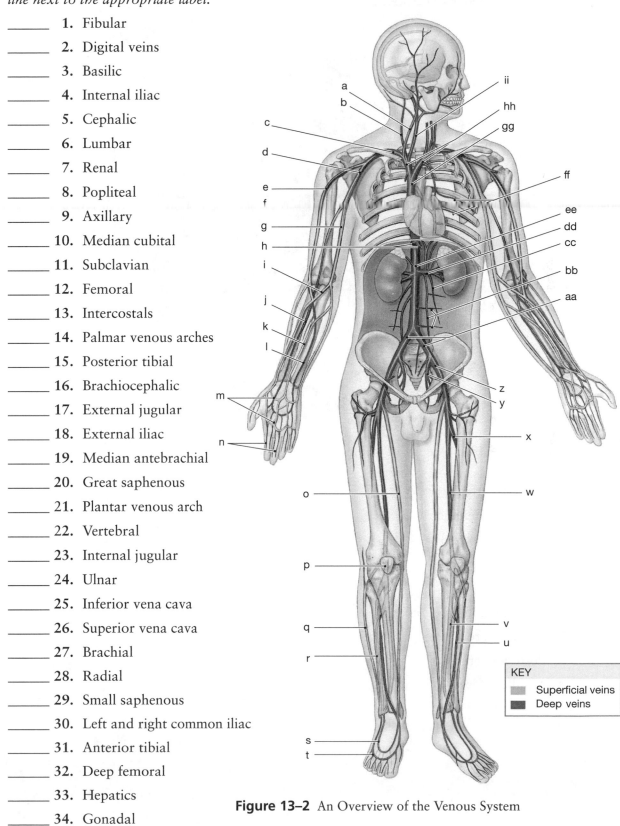

Figure 13–2 An Overview of the Venous System

Identify the arteries of the brain shown in Figure 13–3. Place the corresponding letter on the line next to the appropriate label. <u>Please use each letter only once</u>.

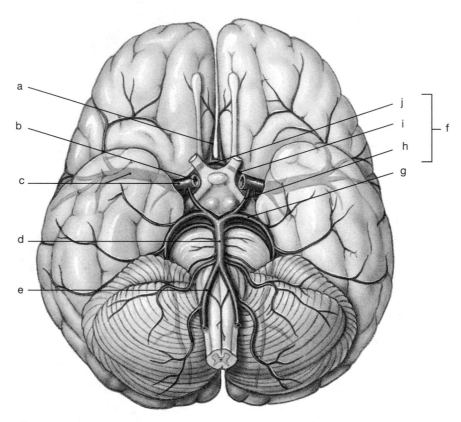

Figure 13–3 Arteries of the Brain

_____ **1.** Cerebral arterial circle

_____ **2.** Anterior communicating

_____ **3.** Anterior cerebral

_____ **4.** Anterior cerebral

_____ **5.** Basilar

_____ **6.** Posterior communicating

_____ **7.** Internal carotid (cut)

_____ **8.** Posterior cerebral

_____ **9.** Middle cerebral

_____ **10.** Vertebral

LABELING EXERCISE 13–4

Identify the major arteries of the trunk shown in Figure 13–4. Place the corresponding letter on the line next to the appropriate label.

_____ 1. Descending aorta (abdominal aorta)

_____ 2. Internal iliac

_____ 3. Suprarenal

_____ 4. Splenic

_____ 5. Pericardial

_____ 6. Intercostals

_____ 7. Diaphragm

_____ 8. Celiac trunk

_____ 9. Bronchials

_____ 10. Thyrocervical trunk

_____ 11. Subclavian

_____ 12. Renal

_____ 13. Common iliac

_____ 14. Phrenics

_____ 15. Inferior mesenteric

_____ 16. Common carotid

_____ 17. Vertebral

_____ 18. Terminal segment of the aorta

_____ 19. Axillary

_____ 20. Descending aorta (thoracic aorta)

_____ 21. Mediastinals

_____ 22. Common hepatic

_____ 23. Left gastric

_____ 24. Lumbar

_____ 25. Internal thoracic

_____ 26. Superior mesenteric

_____ 27. External iliac

_____ 28. Gonadal

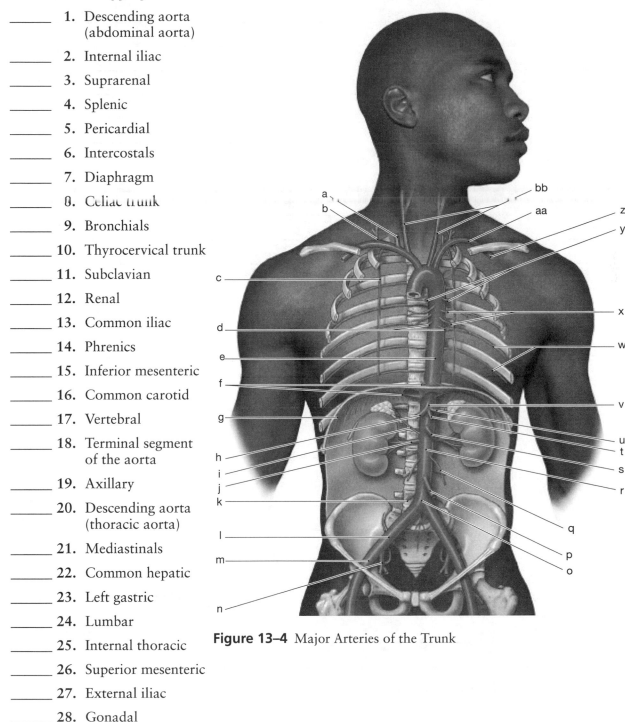

Figure 13–4 Major Arteries of the Trunk

SHORT ANSWER

1. Discuss the three sources of peripheral resistance that are responsible for maintaining blood flow.

   _____

   _____

   _____

   _____

   _____

   _____

2. What occurs inside an artery of someone who has atherosclerosis?

   _____

   _____

   _____

   _____

   _____

3. How does arteriosclerosis affect the structure and function of an artery?

   _____

   _____

   _____

   _____

4. Explain the physiology of an aortic aneurysm.

   _____

   _____

   _____

5. What would happen if the body started to produce too much renin? How would this impact the production of angiotensin II?

   _____

   _____

   _____

   _____

©2008 Pearson Education, Inc.
Anatomy & Physiology for Emergency Care, 2nd ed.

14 The Lymphatic System and Immunity

Chapter Objectives

1. Identify the major components of the lymphatic system and explain their functions.

2. Discuss the importance of lymphocytes and describe where they are found in the body.

3. List the body's nonspecific defenses and explain how each functions.

4. Define specific resistance and identify the forms and properties of immunity.

5. Distinguish between cell-mediated immunity and antibody-mediated (humoral) immunity.

6. Discuss the different types of T cells and the role played by each in the immune response.

7. Describe the structure of antibody molecules and explain how they function.

8. Describe the primary and secondary immune responses to antigen exposure.

9. Relate allergic reactions and autoimmune disorders to immune mechanisms.

10. Describe the changes in the immune system that occur with aging.

11. Discuss the structural and functional interactions between the lymphatic system and other body systems.

Content Self-Evaluation

MULTIPLE CHOICE

_____ 1. The major components of the lymphatic system include the _____.
A. lymphatic vessels
B. lymph
C. lymphocytes
D. All of the above.

_____ 2. Which of the following is *not* made of lymphoidal tissue?
A. tonsils
B. thymus
C. spleen
D. liver

_____ 3. Lymphocytes respond to the presence of _____.
A. invading pathogens
B. cancer cells
C. foreign proteins
D. All of the above.

_____ 4. Lymphatic vessels are structurally similar to _____.
A. arteries
B. capillaries
C. veins
D. arterioles

_____ 5. The three classes of lymphocytes are _____.
A. monocytes, basophils, eosinophils
B. T cells, B cells, NK cells
C. red blood cells, platelets, white blood cells
D. neutrophils, eosinophils, basophils

_____ 6. Lymphocytes account for roughly _____ percent of the circulating white blood cells.
A. 10
B. 15
C. 20
D. 25

_____ 7. The lymphocytes that are responsible for cell-mediated immunity are called _____.
A. NK cells
B. T cells
C. B cells
D. antigens

_____ 8. The lymphocytes that are responsible for the production of antibodies are called _____.
A. T cells
B. B cells
C. NK cells
D. antigens

_____ 9. The lymphocytes that are responsible for attacking foreign cells, including cancer cells, are called _____.
A. B cells
B. T cells
C. NK cells
D. antigens

_____ 10. Hemocytoblasts originate in the bone marrow and produce lymphoid stem cells that produce _____.
A. T cells
B. B cells
C. NK cells
D. All of the above.

_____ 11. A large cluster of lymphoid nodules called a Peyer's patch can be found in the _____.
A. neck
B. inguinal area
C. intestine
D. spleen

_____ 12. Which of the following are responsible for T cell production and maturation?
A. TSH
B. T3
C. T4
D. thymosins

_____ 13. Which of the following is a function of the spleen?
A. removes abnormal red blood cells
B. makes T cells
C. makes B cells
D. stores excess white blood cells

_____ 14. A _____ is an example of a microphage.
   A. lymphocyte   C. monocyte
   B. basophil   D. neutrophil

_____ 15. _____ are macrophage cells found in and around the liver.
   A. Neutrophils   C. Kupffer cells
   B. Eosinophils   D. Cytokines

_____ 16. When NK cells encounter an antigen, it releases a protein that causes the cell to rupture. The name of the protein is _____.
   A. cytokines   C. complement
   B. perforins   D. interferons

_____ 17. Which of the following are small proteins released by lymphocytes that produce antiviral proteins that interfere with viral replication?
   A. cytokines   C. complement
   B. perforins   D. interferons

_____ 18. All of the following are functions of the complement system _except_ _____.
   A. decrease inflammation   C. stimulate phagocytosis
   B. attract phagocytes   D. destroy cell membranes

_____ 19. Circulating proteins that reset the thermostat in the hypothalamus, which causes the body temperature to rise, are called _____.
   A. complement proteins   C. pyrogens
   B. interferons   D. perforins

_____ 20. The specific defense system is activated by contact with a(n) _____.
   A. antibody   C. interferon
   B. antigen   D. pyrogen

_____ 21. The type of immunity that is genetically determined and present at birth is called _____.
   A. active immunity   C. passive immunity
   B. innate immunity   D. acquired immunity

_____ 22. The type of immunity that is produced by the transfer of antibodies to an individual from another source is called _____.
   A. active immunity   C. passive immunity
   B. innate immunity   D. acquired immunity

_____ 23. The use of a vaccine to prevent a certain disease is called _____.
   A. active immunity   C. naturally acquired immunity
   B. innate immunity   D. acquired immunity

_____ 24. The four general properties of the specific defense system include _____.
   A. innate, acquired, passive, active
   B. specificity, versatility, memory, tolerance
   C. interferons, pyrogens, perforins, chemotaxis
   D. inflammation, phagocytosis, fever, physical barriers

_____ 25. The first line of specific defense that occurs with exposure to a pathogen is _____.
   A. B cell activation   C. NK cell activation
   B. phagocytosis   D. T cell activation

_____ 26. Which of the following cells are responsible for cell-mediated immunity?
   A. helper T cells   C. memory T cells
   B. B cells   D. killer T cells

27. Cytotoxic T cells destroy pathogens in all of the following ways *except* _____.
   A. release perforins to rupture target's cell membrane
   B. secrete cytokines that activate pathogen genes to tell them to die
   C. secrete lymphotoxin to disrupt pathogens' metabolism
   D. produce appropriate antibodies

28. Which of the following cells are responsible for immediately differentiating into cytotoxic T cells and helper T cells when the body is exposed to the same antigen the second time?
   A. helper T cells
   B. memory T cells
   C. suppressor T cells
   D. B cells

29. The specificity of the antibody molecule depends on the _____.
   A. size of the antibody
   B. fixed segments of the light and heavy chains
   C. variable segments of the light and heavy chains
   D. size of the antigen

30. All of the following are ways an antibody eliminates antigens *except* _____.
   A. neutralization
   B. activation of complement proteins
   C. agglutination
   D. decreasing inflammation

31. Which of the following is the largest and most diverse of the antibodies?
   A. IgA
   B. IgM
   C. IgG
   D. IgA

32. Which of the following antibodies is responsible for B cell activation?
   A. IgA
   B. IgD
   C. IgE
   D. IgM

33. Which of the following antibodies is responsible for basophil and mast cell release?
   A. IgA
   B. IgE
   C. IgD
   D. IgM

34. Which of the following antibodies is found in exocrine secretions like tears and saliva?
   A. IgA
   B. IgE
   C. IgD
   D. IgM

35. The binding of an antibody to an antigen will result in _____.
   A. neutralizing the antigen
   B. activation of complement system
   C. agglutination
   D. All of the above.

36. The human immunodeficiency virus is a retrovirus that affects which group of cells?
   A. suppressor T cells
   B. memory T cells
   C. B cells
   D. helper T cells

37. _____ are hormones found within the immune system that stimulate the production of neutrophils, eosinophils, and basophils.
   A. Interleukins
   B. Interferons
   C. Tumor necrosis factors
   D. Colony-stimulating factors

38. _____ are hormones found within the immune system that stimulate B cell and antibody production.
   A. Interleukins
   B. Interferons
   C. Tumor necrosis factors
   D. Colony-stimulating factors

39. Misguided antibodies that end up attacking normal cells as if they were antigens are called _____.
   A. allergens
   B. autoantibodies
   C. antigens
   D. mast cells

_____ 40. All of the following are examples of autoimmune diseases *except* _____.
    A. Graves' disease   C. myasthenia gravis
    B. Addison's disease   D. AIDS

_____ 41. Which of the following types of allergies occurs 2 to 3 days after exposure to an antigen?
    A. Type I   C. Type III
    B. Type II   D. Type IV

_____ 42. The type of allergy that is rapid and especially severe in the presence of an antigen is _____.
    A. Type I   C. Type III
    B. Type II   D. Type IV

_____ 43. The type of shock that can occur from a Type I reaction and can lead to life-threatening airway swelling is called _____.
    A. septic shock   C. neurogenic shock
    B. anaphylactic shock   D. toxic shock

_____ 44. _____ is an unexpected and exaggerated reaction to a particular antigen.
    A. Allergy   C. Hypersensitivity
    B. Sensitivity   D. Allergen

_____ 45. The most common cause of fatal anaphylactic reactions is _____.
    A. shellfish   C. penicillin injections
    B. insect bites   D. peanuts

_____ 46. The principle chemical mediator of an allergic reaction is _____.
    A. epinephrine   C. angiotensin
    B. aldosterone   D. histamine

_____ 47. With advancing age, the immune system becomes less effective due to _____.
    A. T cells that are less responsive to antigens
    B. fewer cytotoxic T cells
    C. a reduction in helper T cells
    D. All of the above.

_____ 48. In the elderly, B cells become less active due to a reduced number of _____.
    A. suppressor T cells   C. NK cells
    B. helper T cells   D. antibodies

_____ 49. Signs and symptoms of anaphylaxis typically begin within _____.
    A. 1 to 2 minutes   C. 30 to 60 seconds
    B. 3 to 5 minutes   D. 5 to 10 seconds

_____ 50. All of the following are signs and symptoms of acute anaphylaxis *except* _____.
    A. swelling in the face and neck area   C. wheezing
    B. laryngeal edema   D. relaxation of the bronchioles

FILL IN THE BLANK

1. _____ is the body's ability to resist infection.

2. _____ are responsible for many human diseases.

3. The _____ collects lymph from the lower abdomen, pelvis, and left side of the body.

4. _____ account for roughly 25 percent of circulating white blood cells.

5. Approximately 80 percent of circulating lymphocytes are _____.

6. _____ inhibit both T cells and B cells.

7. _____ make up 10 to 15 percent of circulating lymphocytes.

8. Lymphocyte production and development is called _____.

9. Prior to differentiation, lymphocytes are called _____.

10. The _____ is a pink gland that lies in the mediastinum behind the sternum.

11. _____ stimulate lymphocyte stem cell division and T cell maturation.

12. _____ defenses do not distinguish between one threat or another.

13. _____ defenses protect against particular threats.

14. The first line of cellular defense from a pathogen comes from _____.

15. The process by which antibodies bind to viruses or bacteria making them incapable of attaching to a cell is called _____.

16. _____ are small proteins released by activated lymphocytes, macrophages, and tissue cells infected with viruses.

17. The purposes of inflammation are to allow for _____, _____, and _____.

18. _____ is the tissue destruction that occurs after cells have been injured or destroyed.

19. The _____ are large lymphoid nodules in the walls of the pharynx that guard the entrance to the digestive and respiratory tracts.

20. NK cells secrete proteins called _____ which kill the abnormal cell by creating large pores in its cell membrane.

21. _____ immunity appears after exposure to an antigen as a consequence of the immune response.

22. A mother producing antibodies to protect her baby during gestation is an example of _____ immunity.

23. Class II major histocompatibility complex proteins are found in the membranes of lymphocytes and phagocytes called _____.

24. _____ cells stimulate both cell-mediated immunity and antibody-mediated immunity.

25. _____ cells limit the degree of the immune response.

26. _____ antibodies attack bacteria and are responsible for the cross-reactions between incompatible blood types.

27. _____ antibodies are responsible for stimulating inflammation.

28. The first antibody to appear in the blood is _____.

29. HIV is a retrovirus that carries its genetic information in _____ rather than DNA.

30. _____ slow tumor growth and kill sensitive tumor cells.

31. An active antibody is shaped like the letter _____.

32. _____ hypersensitivity results from cellular immunity and does not involve antibodies.

33. _____ hypersensitivity is a rapid and severe response to the presence of an antigen.

34. An _____ is an exaggerated response by the immune system to a foreign substance.

©2008 Pearson Education, Inc.
Anatomy & Physiology for Emergency Care, 2nd ed.

35. The second most frequent cause of fatal anaphylactic reactions is from _____.

36. _____ develop when the immune response mistakenly targets normal body cells and tissues.

37. In the elderly, T cells become less responsive to _____.

38. Histamine 1 (H1) receptors, when stimulated, will cause _____ and _____.

39. Histamine release from an allergic reaction will cause a rash with raised red bumps. This is called _____.

40. The primary emergency treatment for acute anaphylaxis is _____.

MATCHING

Match the terms in Column A with the words or phrases in Column B. Write the letter of the corresponding words or phrases in the spaces provided.

Column A

_____ 1. graft-versus-host disease

_____ 2. mononucleosis

_____ 3. lymphadenopathy

_____ 4. lymphoma

_____ 5. apoptosis

_____ 6. passive immunity

_____ 7. active immunity

_____ 8. NK cells

_____ 9. B cells

_____ 10. spleen

Column B

a. immunity through breast milk

b. cancer with abnormal lymphocytes

c. immunity through vaccinations

d. largest mass of lymphoidal tissue

e. lymphocyte that stimulates antibody release

f. condition where donor T cells attack recipient tissue

g. enlargement of lymph nodes

h. genetically programmed cell death

i. caused by Epstein-Barr virus

j. lymphocyte that attacks cancer cells

LABELING EXERCISE 14–1

Identify the components of the lymphatic system shown in Figure 14–1. Place the corresponding letter on the line next to the appropriate label.

_____ **1.** Lumbar lymph nodes

_____ **2.** Lymphoid nodules of intestines

_____ **3.** Pelvic lymph nodes

_____ **4.** Right lymphatic duct

_____ **5.** Lymphatics of mammary gland

_____ **6.** Inguinal lymph nodes

_____ **7.** Axillary lymph nodes

_____ **8.** Thymus

_____ **9.** Lymphatics of upper limb

_____ **10.** Lymphatics of lower limb

_____ **11.** Tonsil

_____ **12.** Thoracic (left lymphatic) duct

_____ **13.** Thoracic duct

_____ **14.** Spleen

_____ **15.** Cervical lymph nodes

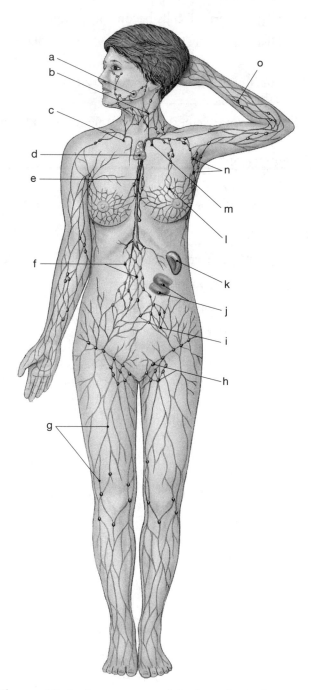

Figure 14–1 Components of the Lymphatic System

©2008 Pearson Education, Inc.
Anatomy & Physiology for Emergency Care, 2nd ed.

LABELING EXERCISE 14–2

Identify the parts of the lymph node shown in Figure 14–2. Place the corresponding letter on the line next to the appropriate label.

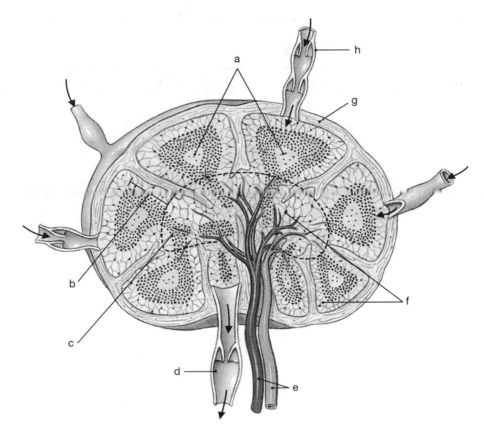

Figure 14–2 The Structure of a Lymph Node

_____ 1. Germinal centers

_____ 2. Medulla

_____ 3. Efferent lymphatic vessel

_____ 4. Afferent lymphatic vessel

_____ 5. Sinuses

_____ 6. Capsule

_____ 7. Lymph node artery and vein

_____ 8. Cortex

SHORT ANSWER

1. What are the differences between active and passive immunity?

_____

_____

_____

_____

2. What are the four types of T cells found in the blood and where do they each originate?

_____

_____

_____

_____

_____

3. What are the three main functions of the lymphatic system?

_____

_____

_____

_____

4. What are the primary functions of B cells and where do they originate?

_____

_____

_____

_____

5. What are the main differences between non-specific and specific defense systems?

_____

_____

_____

_____

15 The Respiratory System

Chapter Objectives

1. Describe the primary functions of the respiratory system. — pp. 547–548

2. Explain how the delicate respiratory exchange surfaces are protected from pathogens, debris, and other hazards. — p. 548

3. Relate respiratory functions to the structural specializations of the tissues and organs in the respiratory system. — pp. 548–560

4. Describe the physical principles that govern the movement of air into the lungs and the diffusion of gases into and out of the blood. — p. 560

5. Describe the actions of respiratory muscles on respiratory movements. — pp. 560–565

6. Describe how oxygen and carbon dioxide are transported in the blood. — pp. 565–572

7. Describe the major factors that influence the rate of respiration. — p. 573

8. Identify the reflexes that regulate respiration. — pp. 574–575, 577

9. Describe the changes that occur in the respiratory system at birth and with aging. — p. 578

10. Discuss the interrelationships between the respiratory system and other systems. — pp. 578–579

Content Self-Evaluation

MULTIPLE CHOICE

_____ 1. Which of the following are functions of the respiratory system?
   A. producing sounds
   B. oxygen and carbon dioxide exchange
   C. protecting the airway surfaces from dehydration
   D. All of the above.

_____ 2. The process of breathing is called _____.
- A. ventilation
- B. pulmonary ventilation
- C. respiration
- D. exhalation

_____ 3. The exchange of carbon dioxide and oxygen takes place in small air sacs within the lungs called _____.
- A. lobes
- B. bronchioles
- C. bronchi
- D. alveoli

_____ 4. Which structure is formed by the palatine and maxillary bones?
- A. soft palate
- B. hard palate
- C. nasopharynx
- D. oral pharynx

_____ 5. All of the following are paranasal sinuses _except_ the _____.
- A. ethmoid sinus
- B. parietal sinus
- C. frontal sinus
- D. sphenoid sinus

_____ 6. Cystic fibrosis is an inherited respiratory disease that involves a defect in the _____.
- A. oral pharynx
- B. nasal pharynx
- C. respiratory mucosa
- D. epiglottis

_____ 7. The movement of carbon dioxide and oxygen in and out of the alveoli occurs by _____.
- A. osmosis
- B. active transport
- C. facilitated transport
- D. diffusion

_____ 8. The shoehorn-shaped _____ prevents liquids or solid food from entering the respiratory tract.
- A. uvula
- B. alveoli
- C. epiglottis
- D. glottis

_____ 9. Most of the anterior and lateral surfaces of the larynx are formed by the _____.
- A. cricoid cartilage
- B. trachea
- C. thyroid cartilage
- D. glottis

_____ 10. The trachea has a C-shaped cartilage structure that protects the airway by _____.
- A. preventing the trachea's collapse or overexpansion
- B. making the tracheal walls stiff
- C. allowing a large mass of food to pass down the esophagus without affecting the airway
- D. All of the above.

_____ 11. Below is a list of structures that are found in the respiratory tree.
- 1. bronchioles
- 2. secondary bronchi
- 3. alveoli
- 4. alveolar ducts
- 5. primary bronchi
- 6. respiratory bronchioles
- 7. terminal bronchioles

Place the above structures in the correct order that air moves through the structures.
- A. 5, 2, 1, 7, 6, 4, 3
- B. 5, 2, 1, 6, 7, 4, 3
- C. 2, 5, 1, 7, 6, 4, 3
- D. 2, 5, 1, 6, 7, 3, 4

_____ 12. During an emergency situation, it is a common occurrence for paramedics to place the endotracheal (ET) tube too far into the trachea so that the ET tube enters the _____.
A. left primary bronchus   C. carina
B. right primary bronchus   D. left secondary bronchi

_____ 13. The bronchioles within the respiratory system dilate and constrict based on influence from the autonomic nervous system. Stimulation of the sympathetic nervous system causes _____.
A. bronchiole constriction   C. alveolar constriction
B. bronchodilation   D. alveolar dilation

_____ 14. Bronchiolitis is an infection of the smaller airways and is typically seen in children _____.
A. between 2 and 6 months of age   C. between 4 and 6 years old
B. less than 2 years of age   D. between 6 and 10 years old

_____ 15. The alveolar epithelium is primarily comprised of _____ epithelial cells.
A. squamous   C. columnar
B. cuboidal   D. transitional

_____ 16. Dust cells found within the epithelium of the alveoli are responsible for phagocytizing dust or debris found on the alveolar surface. These dust cells are _____.
A. alveolar NK cells   C. cytotoxic cells
B. alveolar macrophages   D. B cells

_____ 17. Surfactant is an oily secretion found within the alveoli that is responsible for _____.
A. increasing surface tension in the alveoli
B. increasing the surface area of the alveoli
C. reducing the air-water boundary and reducing the surface tension in the alveoli
D. increasing the air-water boundary and increasing the surface tension in the alveoli

_____ 18. Which of the following cells produces surfactant?
A. alveoli   C. chief cells
B. septal cells   D. parietal cells

_____ 19. The respiratory membrane consists of all of the following components *except* the _____.
A. squamous epithelium
B. endothelial cells that line an adjacent capillary
C. interstitial membrane that separates the alveoli from the capillary
D. surfactant

_____ 20. Pulmonary embolisms are blood clots that travel and lodge within the pulmonary circulation. All of the following are causes for pulmonary embolisms *except* _____.
A. deep vein thrombosis   C. long plane ride
B. acute arterial occlusion   D. prolonged immobilization

_____ 21. The term used to describe low tissue oxygen levels is _____.
A. anoxia   C. hypoxia
B. acidosis   D. hypocarbia

_____ 22. All of the following are steps in the process of respiration *except* _____.
A. pulmonary ventilation
B. oxygen and carbon dioxide transport
C. oxygen and carbon dioxide exchange
D. oxygenated blood transported to left atrium

_____ 23. The normal tidal volume setting on a ventilator is typically _____.
A. 5–10 mL/kg   C. 15–20 mL/kg
B. 10–15 mL/kg   D. 20–25 mL/kg

_____ 24. The FiO$_2$ setting on a ventilator represents the _____.
     A. inspired oxygen concentration   C. vital capacity
     B. tidal volume   D. respiratory reserve

_____ 25. The most common complication when using a mechanical ventilator with positive-end expiratory pressure is _____.
     A. pneumothorax   C. oxygen toxicity
     B. pneumonia   D. decrease in cardiac output

_____ 26. The movement of air in and out of the lungs is dependent upon _____.
     A. pressure differences between the lungs and the atmosphere
     B. pressure differences between the diaphragm and the pleural space
     C. pressure differences between the capillaries and alveoli
     D. pressure differences between the atmosphere and the inspiratory reserve volume

_____ 27. During exhalation, the diaphragm moves _____.
     A. upward and the ribs move downward
     B. downward and the ribs move downward
     C. upward and the ribs move upward
     D. downward and the ribs move upward

_____ 28. During inspiration, a(n) _____ occurs.
     A. decrease in intrapulmonary pressure   C. increase in intrapulmonary pressure
     B. increase in atmospheric pressure   D. decrease in atmospheric pressure

_____ 29. The maximum amount of air that can move in and out of the lungs in one single respiration is called the _____.
     A. tidal volume   C. inspiratory reserve
     B. vital capacity   D. expiratory reserve

_____ 30. The amount of air that remains in your lungs after maximal expiration is called the _____.
     A. vital capacity   C. residual volume
     B. expiratory reserve   D. minimal volume

_____ 31. The amount of air that can be taken in over and above the resting tidal volume is called the _____.
     A. expiratory reserve volume   C. tidal volume
     B. inspiratory reserve volume   D. vital capacity

_____ 32. Status asthmaticus is a severe, prolonged attack that does not respond to _____.
     A. oxygen   C. intubation
     B. bronchodilators   D. All of the above.

_____ 33. A respiratory disease that is caused by an acute bronchospasm and inflammatory disorder is called _____.
     A. emphysema   C. asthma
     B. chronic bronchitis   D. pneumothorax

_____ 34. Which of the following respiratory diseases are usually caused by cigarette smoking?
     A. asthma   C. emphysema
     B. chronic bronchitis   D. chronic bronchitis and emphysema

_____ 35. Which of the following respiratory diseases leads to pulmonary hypertension and right-sided heart failure?
     A. asthma   C. chronic bronchitis
     B. emphysema   D. pneumonia

_____ 36. Which of the following respiratory diseases results from an increase in the number of goblet cells in the respiratory tree?
A. asthma
B. emphysema
C. chronic bronchitis
D. pneumonia

_____ 37. What is the percentage of oxygen that is carried by the hemoglobin in the red blood cells?
A. 10 percent
B. 50.5 percent
C. 98.5 percent
D. 100 percent

_____ 38. The use of pulse oximetry (SpO_2) is very common in medicine today. Pulse oximetry measures _____.
A. carbon dioxide saturation
B. venous oxygen levels
C. hemoglobin oxygen saturation
D. carbon dioxide levels

_____ 39. Because of the chemical structure of the molecule, _____ has more than 200 times the affinity of oxygen to bind with hemoglobin.
A. carbon dioxide
B. carbon tetrachloride
C. carbon monoxide
D. nitrogen

_____ 40. Most of the carbon dioxide that is transported in the blood is in the form of _____.
A. carbonic acid
B. carbon dioxide
C. bicarbonate ions
D. carbaminohemoglobin

_____ 41. The involuntary respiratory centers of the brain are located within the _____.
A. cerebrum and cerebellum
B. pons and medulla oblongata
C. cerebrum and brainstem
D. hippocampus and midbrain

_____ 42. Which of the following has the greatest impact on the respiratory center of the brain under normal situations?
A. decrease in Po_2
B. increase and decrease in Pco_2
C. increase and decrease in Po_2 and Pco_2
D. increase in Po_2

_____ 43. In a normal healthy adult, the drive to breathe is based on a change in _____ levels in the blood.
A. oxygen
B. nitrogen
C. carbon dioxide
D. hemoglobin

_____ 44. _____ refers to a rise in carbon dioxide levels in the blood.
A. Hypocapnia
B. Hypercapnia
C. Hypoxia
D. Anoxia

_____ 45. In cases of certain advanced respiratory diseases, the desire to breathe is based on _____ levels, not _____ levels.
A. carbon dioxide, oxygen
B. oxygen, carbon dioxide
C. nitrogen, oxygen
D. oxygen, nitrogen

_____ 46. A capnograph is a monitoring device that measures the level of _____.
A. oxygen levels during inhalation
B. carbon dioxide levels during inhalation
C. oxygen levels during exhalation
D. carbon dioxide levels during exhalation

_____ 47. The basic pace of respiration is controlled by all of the following receptors _except_

_____.
A. chemoreceptors
B. stretch receptors
C. proprioreceptors
D. baroreceptors

_____ 48. Before the delivery of an infant, all of the following are true _except_ _____.
A. the pulmonary vessels are dilated due to low pressure
B. the pulmonary vessels are constricted
C. the rib cage is compressed
D. most of the respiratory system contains fluid with no oxygen present

_____ 49. With aging comes an increase in stiffness of the chest wall and a reduction in pulmonary ventilation. This has the greatest impact on _____.
   A. tidal volume   C. residual volume
   B. vital capacity   D. inspiratory reserve

_____ 50. The biggest cause of a reduction in chest movement in the elderly is caused by _____.
   A. smoking   C. emphysema
   B. arthritic changes in the rib cage   D. pneumonia

FILL IN THE BLANK

1. Air normally enters the respiratory system through the paired _____ .

2. _____ monitoring is a noninvasive method of measuring the levels of carbon dioxide in the exhaled breath.

3. Air enters the larynx through a narrow opening called the _____.

4. The shoehorn-shaped _____ projects above the glottis.

5. The anterior surface of the thyroid cartilage forms the _____.

6. The walls of the trachea are supported by _____.

7. The right and left primary bronchi branch into _____.

8. Parasympathetic stimulation leads to _____ of the airway.

9. Respiratory bronchioles open into passages called _____.

10. _____ is the sudden death of an infant under the age of one year that remains unexplained after autopsy.

11. Within the thoracic cavity are two cavities that each contain one lung. This cavity is surrounded by a serous membrane called the _____.

12. When blood accumulates within the pleural cavity, this is called a _____.

13. _____ is the term used when oxygen is completely cut off from the tissues.

14. _____ is the pressure within the airway at the end of expiration.

15. The amount of air that moves in and out of the lungs during a normal respiration is called _____.

16. The amount of air that can be voluntarily expelled at the end of a respiration is called the _____.

17. Oxygen molecules comprise _____ of the atmospheric content of gases.

18. _____ is a disease that results from destruction of the alveolar walls.

19. _____ is a chronic inflammatory disease of the airway.

20. Roughly _____ percent of the oxygen content in the arterial blood is bound to hemoglobin.

21. In active tissues found in the body, normally hemoglobin will release up to _____ percent of the stored oxygen in the hemoglobin.

22. About 70 percent of all carbon dioxide in the body is transported in the plasma as _____.

23. An elevated body temperature will cause respirations to _____.

24. Central nervous system depressants will cause respirations to _____.

25. The _____ prevents the lungs from overexpanding during forced breathing.

MATCHING

Match the terms in Column A with the words or phrases in Column B. Write the letter of the corresponding words or phrases in the spaces provided.

Column A

_____ 1. dyspnea

_____ 2. apnea

_____ 3. epistaxis

_____ 4. tidal volume

_____ 5. respiratory distress syndrome

_____ 6. pleurisy

_____ 7. atelectasis

_____ 8. anoxia

_____ 9. thyroid cartilage

_____ 10. FiO$_2$

Column B

a. normal inhalation and exhalation

b. inadequate surfactant production

c. collapsed lung

d. cessation of breathing

e. difficult breathing

f. lack of oxygen in the tissues

g. inspired oxygen concentration

h. nose bleed

i. inflammation of the pleura

j. Adam's apple

LABELING EXERCISE 15–1

Identify the components of the respiratory system shown in Figure 15–1. Place the corresponding letter on the line next to the appropriate label.

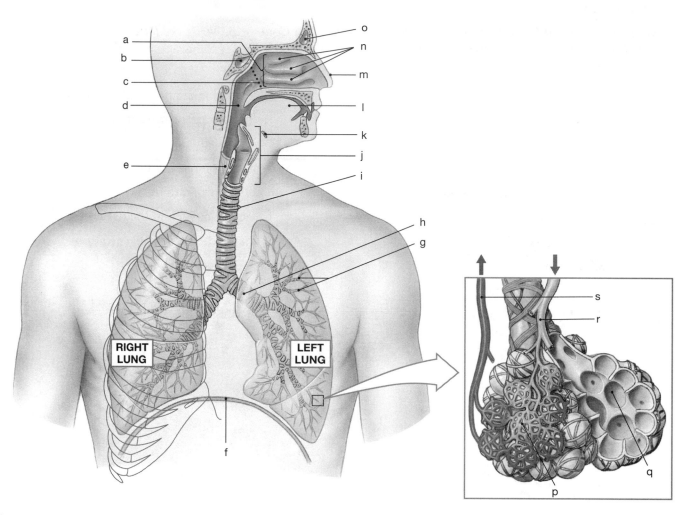

Figure 15–1 Components of the Respiratory System

_____ 1. Bronchioles

_____ 2. Trachea

_____ 3. Nasal conchae

_____ 4. Pharynx

_____ 5. Capillary network

_____ 6. Tongue

_____ 7. Sphenoidal sinus

_____ 8. Hyoid bone

_____ 9. Artery

_____ 10. Nasal cavity

_____ 11. Vein

_____ 12. Diaphragm

_____ 13. Larynx

_____ 14. Alveolus

_____ 15. Internal nares

_____ 16. Frontal sinus

_____ 17. Esophagus

_____ 18. Nose

_____ 19. Bronchus

©2008 Pearson Education, Inc.
Anatomy & Physiology for Emergency Care, 2nd ed.

LABELING EXERCISE 15–2

Identify the structures of the nasal cavity and pharynx shown in Figure 15–2. Place the corresponding letter on the line next to the appropriate label.

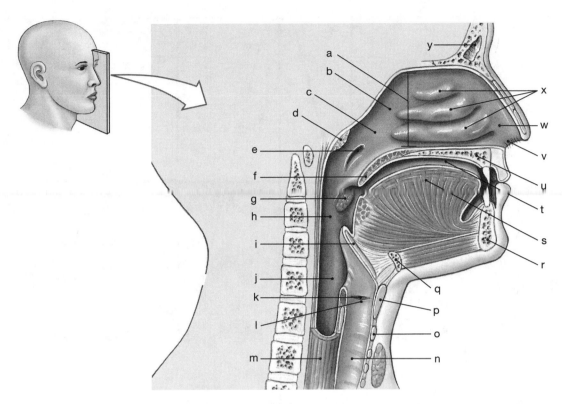

Figure 15–2 The Nose, Nasal Cavity, and Pharynx

_____ 1. Cricoid cartilage

_____ 2. Pharyngeal tonsil

_____ 3. Hyoid bone

_____ 4. Laryngopharynx

_____ 5. Tongue

_____ 6. Soft palate

_____ 7. Hard palate

_____ 8. Vocal fold

_____ 9. Frontal sinus

_____ 10. Internal nares

_____ 11. Nasal vestibule

_____ 12. Oropharynx

_____ 13. Trachea

_____ 14. External nares

_____ 15. Entrance to auditory tube

_____ 16. Nasal conchae

_____ 17. Epiglottis

_____ 18. Glottis

_____ 19. Oral cavity

_____ 20. Nasal cavity

_____ 21. Mandible

_____ 22. Palatine tonsil

_____ 23. Esophagus

_____ 24. Thyroid cartilage

_____ 25. Nasopharynx

LABELING EXERCISE 15–3

Identify the respiratory volumes and capacities shown in Figure 15–3. Place the corresponding letter on the line next to the appropriate label.

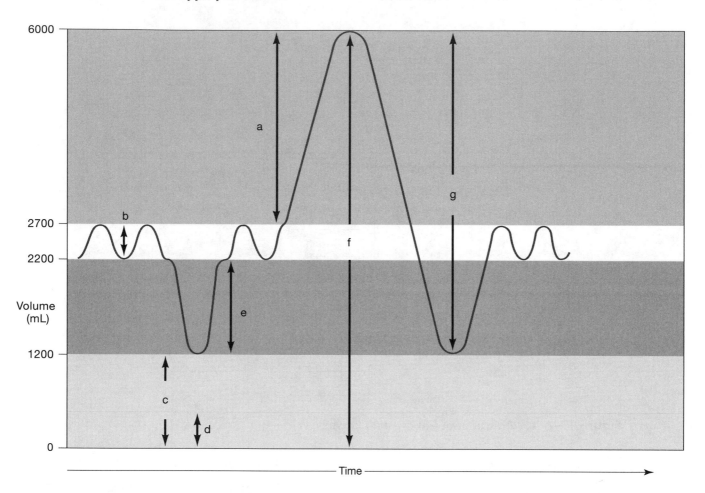

Figure 15–3 Respiratory Volumes and Capacities

_____ **1.** Residual volume

_____ **2.** Expiratory reserve volume

_____ **3.** Total lung capacity

_____ **4.** Inspiratory reserve volume

_____ **5.** Minimal volume

_____ **6.** Vital capacity

_____ **7.** Tidal volume

SHORT ANSWER

1. What are the five functions of the respiratory system?

   _____

   _____

   _____

   _____

   _____

2. Describe the disease asthma and list the factors that are associated with causing an attack.

   _____

   _____

   _____

   _____

   _____

3. What is vital capacity and how do you calculate it?

   _____

   _____

   _____

   _____

   _____

4. What are the three methods by which the body transports carbon dioxide in the blood?

   _____

   _____

   _____

   _____

5. Describe the disease emphysema and name the major contributor that causes the disease.

   _____

   _____

   _____

   _____

   _____

16 The Digestive System

Chapter Objectives

Content Self-Evaluation

MULTIPLE CHOICE

_____ 1. The digestive tract has four major layers: mucosa, submucosa, muscularis externa, and _____.
   A. muscularis interna   C. muscularis intima
   B. serosa   D. lamina propia

_____ 2. Which of the following abdominal organs does *not* assist in the digestive process?
   A. pancreas   C. liver
   B. gallbladder   D. spleen

_____ 3. Which of the following is the normal path that food takes through the digestive tract?
   A. oral cavity, esophagus, stomach, pharynx, large intestine, small intestine, anus, rectum
   B. oral cavity, pharynx, esophagus, stomach, small intestine, large intestine, rectum, anus
   C. pharynx, oral cavity, esophagus, stomach, small intestine, large intestine, rectum, anus
   D. pharynx, oral cavity, esophagus, stomach, large intestine, small intestine, rectum, anus

_____ 4. The part of the intestine that is responsible for controlling and coordinating contractions of the smooth muscle is located in the _____.
   A. mucosa   C. muscularis externa
   B. submucosa   D. serosa

_____ 5. The _____ covers the muscularis externa along most portions of the digestive tract within the peritoneal cavity.
   A. serosa   C. adventitia
   B. submucosa   D. intima

_____ 6. The network of nerves that is responsible for sympathetic and parasympathetic functions is located in the _____.
   A. submucosa   C. muscularis externa
   B. mucosa   D. villa

_____ 7. Most of the digestive tract is lined with _____.
   A. stratified squamous epithelium   C. cuboidal epithelium
   B. simple columnar epithelium   D. simple squamous epithelium

_____ 8. The type of epithelial tissue found in the oral cavity, esophagus, and anus is called _____.
   A. simple squamous epithelium   C. simple columnar epithelium
   B. cuboidal epithelium   D. stratified squamous epithelium

_____ 9. The process of using waves of muscular contraction to propel material from one part of the digestive tract to another is called _____.
   A. segmentation   C. ascites
   B. peristalsis   D. contraction

_____ 10. Functions of the oral cavity include _____.
   A. mechanical processing
   B. begins the digestion of carbohydrates and lipids with salivary enzymes
   C. lubricates material by mixing it with mucus and saliva
   D. All of the above.

_____ 11. The cranial nerve that innervates the tongue is the _____ nerve.
   A. abducens   C. trochlear
   B. facial   D. glossopharyngeal

©2008 Pearson Education, Inc.
Anatomy & Physiology for Emergency Care, 2nd ed.

_____ 12. A function of the tongue is _____.
  A. the mechanical processing of food
  B. the sensory analysis of food
  C. manipulating food in the mouth to assist in chewing
  D. All of the above.

_____ 13. There are three pairs of salivary glands that secrete fluid into the oral cavity. Which of the following is *not* an example of a salivary gland?
  A. parotid   C. submandibular
  B. sublingual   D. subpalatine

_____ 14. Salivary amylase released by the salivary glands helps to digest _____.
  A. carbohydrates   C. lipids
  B. fats   D. proteins

_____ 15. Salivary secretions are normally controlled by the _____.
  A. hypothalamus   C. midbrain
  B. autonomic nervous system   D. reticular activating system

_____ 16. The bulk of each tooth consists of _____.
  A. a pulp cavity   C. dentin
  B. a root canal   D. enamel

_____ 17. During the process of swallowing, all of the following actions occur *except* the _____.
  A. epiglottis folds   C. soft palate moves upward
  B. larynx moves upward   D. glottis opens up

_____ 18. The smallest part of the stomach is called the _____.
  A. fundus   C. pylorus
  B. cardia   D. body

_____ 19. The _____ regulates the flow of chyme between the stomach and the small intestine.
  A. fundus   C. pyloric sphincter
  B. cardia   D. rugae

_____ 20. The ridges and folds found within the stomach provide a greater surface area for the breakdown of food. This area is called the _____.
  A. pylorus   C. greater omentum
  B. rugae   D. gastric pits

_____ 21. Hydrochloric acid lowers the pH of the stomach contents. Which of the following cells is responsible for secreting the hydrochloric acid?
  A. gastric pits   C. chief cells
  B. parietal cells   D. gastric glands

_____ 22. _____ secrete(s) pepsinogen into the stomach lumen to help break down proteins.
  A. Chief cells   C. Parietal cells
  B. Gastric pits   D. Rennin

_____ 23. The bacteria _____ was found in approximately 80 percent of all cases of gastric and duodenal ulcers. Aggressive treatment has helped to eradicate the bacteria and decrease the incidence of peptic disease.
  A. *Staphylococcus aureus*   C. *Helicobacter pylori*
  B. *Streptococcus pyogenes*   D. *Streptococcus epidermidis*

_____ 24. The phase that is initiated by the sight, smell, or taste of food is called the _____.
  A. gastric phase   C. cephalic phase
  B. intestinal phase   D. bowel phase

_____ 25. _____ is an endocrine hormone released from the gastric glands in the stomach to help churn or mix gastric contents.
A. Secretin
B. Cholecystokinin
C. Gastrin
D. Pepsin

_____ 26. Which of the following is the correct order of swallowing phases?
A. oral, esophageal, pharyngeal
B. oral, pharyngeal, esophageal
C. pharyngeal, oral, esophageal
D. pharyngeal, esophageal, oral

_____ 27. The common name for backflow of stomach contents toward the esophagus is _____.
A. esophagitis
B. a hernia
C. heartburn
D. an ulcer

_____ 28. The phase where the chyme begins to enter the duodenum is called the _____.
A. gastric phase
B. duodenal phase
C. intestinal phase
D. cephalic phase

_____ 29. All of the following statements are true regarding why there is a limited amount of digestion that occurs in the stomach _except_:
A. the epithelial cells are covered by a blanket of acidic mucus and are not directly exposed to chyme.
B. the epithelial cells lack the specialized transport mechanisms normally found in cells lining the small intestine.
C. the gastric lining is impermeable to water.
D. digestion is not completed in the stomach because most carbohydrates, fats, and proteins have only been partially broken down.

_____ 30. Which of the following is the correct order that chyme travels through the small intestine?
A. ileum, jejunum, duodenum
B. jejunum, ileum, duodenum
C. duodenum, jejunum, ileum
D. jejunum, duodenum, ileum

_____ 31. A gastrointestinal (GI) bleed is considered to be in the upper portion of the GI tract when it is proximal to the _____.
A. stomach
B. large intestine
C. ligament of Treitz
D. esophageal ligament

_____ 32. Regional movements of the muscle that churn and fragment the digestive material is called _____.
A. mastication
B. peristalsis
C. segmentation
D. defecation

_____ 33. The valve that connects the small and large intestine is called the _____.
A. appendix
B. ileointestinal valve
C. ileocecal valve
D. sigmoidal valve

_____ 34. Nutrients from the small intestine enter the bloodstream through a network of projections called _____.
A. plicae
B. gastric pits
C. lacteals
D. villi

_____ 35. The majority of the absorption of nutrients occurs in what part of the small intestine?
A. cecum
B. ileum
C. duodenum
D. jejunum

_____ 36. The hormone that stimulates the release of insulin into the blood when glucose is present is called_____.
A. gastrin
B. secretin
C. cholecystokinin (CCK)
D. gastric inhibitory peptide (GIP)

©2008 Pearson Education, Inc.
Anatomy & Physiology for Emergency Care, 2nd ed.

37. Which of the following is the hormone that stimulates the gallbladder to release bile?
   A. gastrin
   B. secretin
   C. cholecystokinin (CCK)
   D. gastric inhibitory peptide (GIP)

38. The intestinal hormone that stimulates the pancreas to release bicarbonate ions is called _____.
   A. gastrin
   B. secretin
   C. bile
   D. cholecystokinin

39. _____ is a hormone that stimulates chief cells and parietal cells in the stomach.
   A. Cholecystokinin
   B. Gastrin
   C. Secretin
   D. Gastric inhibitory peptide

40. The pancreas is an essential organ when it comes to digestion. Not only does it release insulin and glucagon, but it also releases _____ to aid in digestion.
   A. lipases
   B. pancreatic amylase
   C. proteases
   D. All of the above.

41. Within the pancreas, the pancreatic islets are responsible for producing _____.
   A. carbohydrases
   B. glucagon
   C. insulin
   D. All of the above.

42. Which of the following is the most common cause of portal hypertension?
   A. splenomegaly
   B. cirrhosis
   C. pancreatitis
   D. gallbladder disease

43. The three segments of the large intestine are _____.
   A. duodenum, ileum, jejunum
   B. sigmoid colon, anus, rectum
   C. ascending, transverse, descending
   D. ileocecum, colon, anus

44. Which of the following organs is responsible for storage of glycogen?
   A. pancreas
   B. liver
   C. gallbladder
   D. appendix

45. Which of the following forms of hepatitis is most commonly transmitted via the fecal/oral route?
   A. hepatitis A
   B. hepatitis B
   C. hepatitis C
   D. hepatitis D

46. Which of the following forms of hepatitis is transmitted via blood, saliva, or semen?
   A. hepatitis A
   B. hepatitis B
   C. hepatitis E
   D. hepatitis D

47. Bacteria within the large intestine produce an important vitamin that assists with glucose metabolism. The vitamin is called _____.
   A. thiamine
   B. biotin
   C. pantothenic acid
   D. niacin

48. One of the main functions of the large intestine is to _____.
   A. absorb carbohydrates and fats
   B. absorb amino acids
   C. absorb water
   D. breakdown remaining food material

49. Which of the following vitamins is necessary for blood coagulation, and is deficient in the presence of chronic liver failure?
   A. vitamin D
   B. vitamin K
   C. vitamin A
   D. vitamin B-12

50. Which of the following forms of cancer are more common in the elderly who smoke?
   A. lung and liver
   B. colon and lung
   C. oral and pharyngeal
   D. skin and liver

FILL IN THE BLANK

1. The _____ is the inner lining of the digestive tract.

2. The _____ layer of the intestinal wall contains large blood vessels and parasympathetic motor neurons.

3. The muscularis externa propels food from one part of the digestive tract to the other by way of _____.

4. The mechanical mixing of the food in the digestive tract is called _____.

5. _____ is an enzyme that breaks down complex carbohydrates into smaller molecules.

6. Each tooth consists of a mineralized matrix similar to bone called _____.

7. The _____ is the common passageway for food.

8. The _____ is a muscular tube approximately 10 inches long that transports food to the stomach.

9. The other term for swallowing is _____.

10. A weakened esophageal sphincter can cause _____, which is a type of inflammation.

11. Ingested food that has turned into a soupy mixture is called _____.

12. _____ is the accumulation of fluid in the peritoneal cavity.

13. _____ is a condition caused by bacterial toxins, viral infections, or various poisons and characterized by vomiting and diarrhea.

14. The stomach is lined by a _____ epithelium that is dominated by mucous cells.

15. Each day gastric glands secrete about _____ of gastric juice into the stomach.

16. Parietal cells in the stomach secrete _____ and _____.

17. Newborn babies produce _____ to coagulate the milk to slow digestion.

18. _____ are erosions in the stomach caused by gastric acid.

19. The _____ phase is when the chyme moves from the stomach to the small intestine.

20. The _____ plays a key role in the digestion and absorption of nutrients.

21. The transverse folds within the intestinal wall are called _____.

22. _____ is the neurotransmitter that is released from the lining of the intestinal wall and from neurons in the brain that stimulate vomiting.

23. _____ is released when the pH decreases in the duodenum.

24. _____ is released when fats and carbohydrates enter the small intestine.

25. _____ is released in the duodenum in response to a large quantity of incompletely digested proteins.

26. As chyme begins to enter the duodenum, _____ is released to increase bile in the duodenum.

27. The right and left lobes of the liver are divided by a tough connective tissue called the _____.

28. The phagocytic cells found within the liver are called _____.

29. Bile released from the gallbladder is responsible for the _____ of fats.

©2008 Pearson Education, Inc.
Anatomy & Physiology for Emergency Care, 2nd ed.

30. The most common cause of chronic viral hepatitis in the Unites States is _____.

31. The main function of the gallbladder is _____.

32. The most common location of abdominal pain in the case of an acute gallbladder attack is the _____.

33. The appendix primarily functions as an organ of the _____ system.

34. The feature of the large intestine that makes it look differently than the rest of the intestine is the presence of large pouches called _____.

35. Three longitudinal bands of smooth muscle called _____ run along the outside of the colon beneath the serosa.

36. Vitamin K is a fat-soluble vitamin needed by the liver to synthesize the clotting factor _____.

37. Digestive enzymes break bonds between molecules in a process called _____.

38. Vitamin _____ is an essential vitamin in the first step of Kreb's cycle and for other metabolic processes.

39. In the elderly, a decrease in the motility of the intestinal tract leads to _____.

40. _____ is a disease that is characterized by widespread destruction of hepatocytes.

MATCHING

Match the terms in Column A with the words or phrases in Column B. Write the letter of the corresponding words or phrases in the spaces provided.

Column A

_____ 1. peritonitis

_____ 2. polyps

_____ 3. ascites

_____ 4. inflammatory bowel disease

_____ 5. mastication

_____ 6. chyme

_____ 7. pepsin

_____ 8. gastrectomy

_____ 9. achalasia

_____ 10. colectomy

Column B

a. accumulation of fluid in the abdomen

b. chewing

c. proteolytic enzyme

d. removal of all or a portion of the colon

e. mucosal tumors

f. inflammation of the peritoneal membrane

g. bolus cannot reach stomach due to a constriction of the esophagus

h. chronic inflammation of the digestive tract

i. partially digested food

j. surgical removal of stomach

Identify the components of the digestive system shown in Figure 16–1. Place the corresponding letter on the line next to the appropriate label.

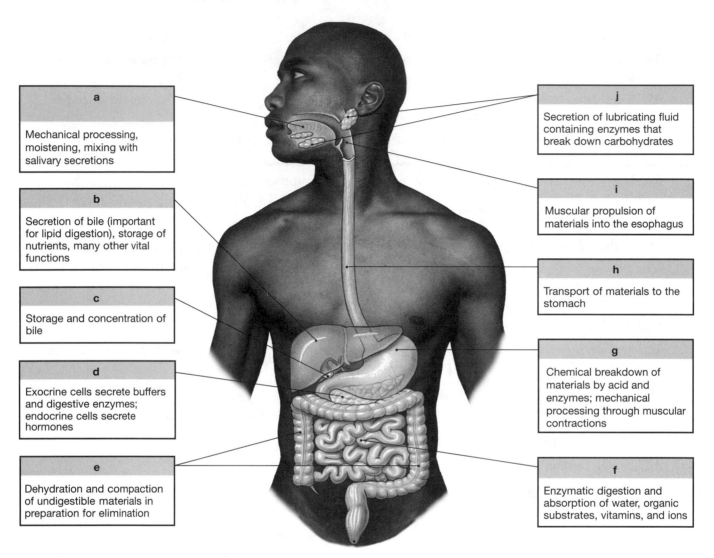

a

Mechanical processing, moistening, mixing with salivary secretions

b

Secretion of bile (important for lipid digestion), storage of nutrients, many other vital functions

c

Storage and concentration of bile

d

Exocrine cells secrete buffers and digestive enzymes; endocrine cells secrete hormones

e

Dehydration and compaction of undigestible materials in preparation for elimination

j

Secretion of lubricating fluid containing enzymes that break down carbohydrates

i

Muscular propulsion of materials into the esophagus

h

Transport of materials to the stomach

g

Chemical breakdown of materials by acid and enzymes; mechanical processing through muscular contractions

f

Enzymatic digestion and absorption of water, organic substrates, vitamins, and ions

Figure 16–1 Components of the Digestive System

_____ 1. Pharynx

_____ 2. Gallbladder

_____ 3. Small intestine

_____ 4. Esophagus

_____ 5. Oral cavity teeth, tongue

_____ 6. Pancreas

_____ 7. Liver

_____ 8. Salivary glands

_____ 9. Stomach

_____ 10. Large intestine

LABELING EXERCISE 16–2

Identify the parts of the digestive tract shown in Figure 16–2. Place the corresponding letter on the line next to the appropriate label.

_____ 1. Muscularis externa

_____ 2. Mucosa

_____ 3. Mesentery

_____ 4. Plicae

_____ 5. Submucosa

_____ 6. Mesenteric artery and vein

_____ 7. Serosa (visceral peritoneum)

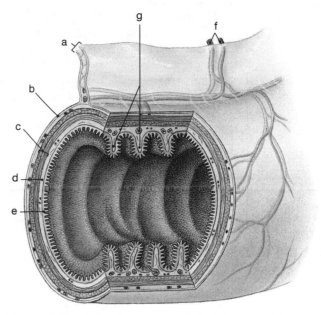

Figure 16–2 The Structure of the Digestive Tract

LABELING EXERCISE 16–3

Identify the parts of the digestive tract shown in Figure 16–3. Place the corresponding letter on the line next to the appropriate label. _Please use each letter only once._

_____ 1. Submucosa

_____ 2. Submucosal plexus

_____ 3. Submucosal gland

_____ 4. Mucous epithelium

_____ 5. Artery and vein

_____ 6. Muscularis mucosae

_____ 7. Villi

_____ 8. Mucosa

_____ 9. Muscularis externa

_____ 10. Plica

_____ 11. Myenteric plexus

_____ 12. Mucosal glands

_____ 13. Lymphatic vessel

_____ 14. Mucosa

_____ 15. Lamina propria

_____ 16. Serosa (visceral peritoneum)

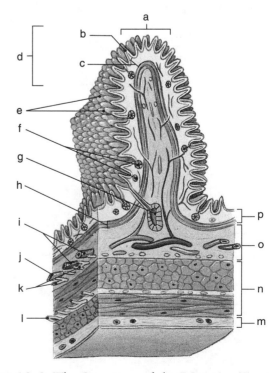

Figure 16–3 The Structure of the Digestive Tract

LABELING EXERCISE 16–4

Identify the superficial landmarks of the stomach shown in Figure 16–4. Place the corresponding letter on the line next to the appropriate label.

_____ 1. Lesser curvature (medial surface)

_____ 2. Rugae

_____ 3. Greater curvature (lateral surface)

_____ 4. Esophagus

_____ 5. Greater omentum

_____ 6. Cardia

_____ 7. Diaphragm

_____ 8. Pylorus

_____ 9. Fundus

_____ 10. Body

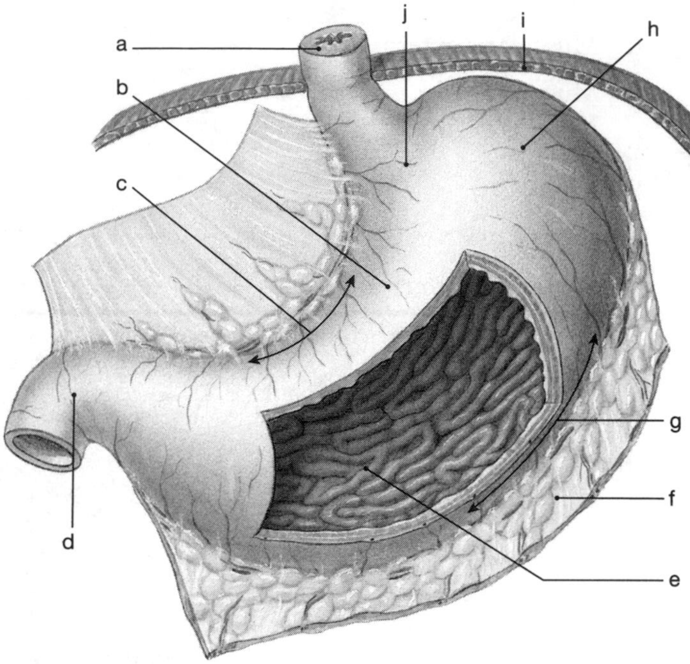

Figure 16–4 Anatomy of the Stomach

LABELING EXERCISE 16–5

Identify the parts of the large intestine shown in Figure 16–5. Place the corresponding letter on the line next to the appropriate label.

_____ 1. Anus

_____ 2. Anal columns

_____ 3. Superior mesenteric vein

_____ 4. Descending colon

_____ 5. Taenia coli

_____ 6. Rectum

_____ 7. Aorta

_____ 8. Inferior mesenteric artery

_____ 9. Greater omentum (cut)

_____ 10. Superior mesenteric artery

_____ 11. Vermiform appendix

_____ 12. Transverse colon

_____ 13. Haustra

_____ 14. External anal sphincter

_____ 15. Inferior mesenteric vein

_____ 16. Ileocecal valve

_____ 17. Sigmoid colon

_____ 18. Splenic vein

_____ 19. Inferior vena cava

_____ 20. Ascending colon

_____ 21. Anal canal

_____ 22. Cecum

_____ 23. Internal anal sphincter

_____ 24. Hepatic portal vein

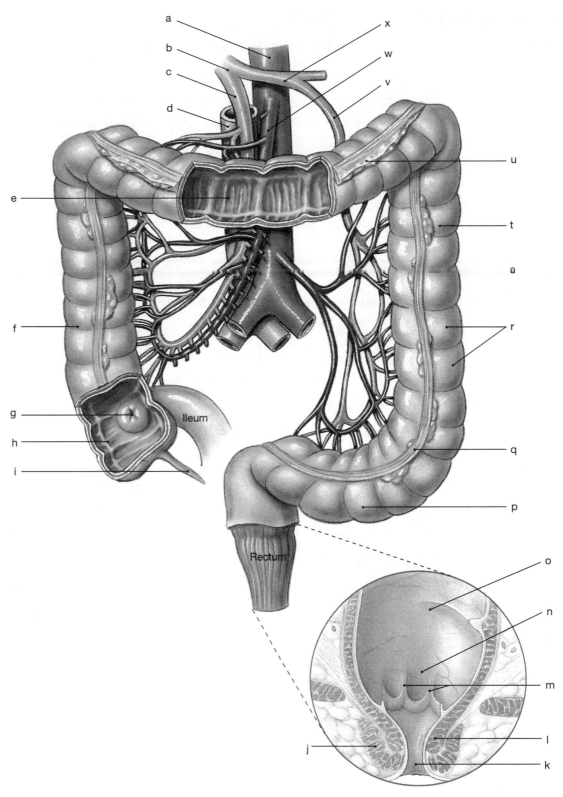

Figure 16–5 Anatomy of the Large Intestine

SHORT ANSWER

1. Compare parietal cells and chief cells and their effects on digestion.

   _____

   _____

   _____

   _____

2. Name and discuss the four intestinal hormones that aid in digestion.

   _____

   _____

   _____

   _____

3. Discuss what causes the majority of peptic ulcers and how they are treated.

   _____

   _____

   _____

   _____

4. Describe the Mallory-Weiss syndrome and its clinical significance.

   _____

   _____

   _____

   _____

5. List the three phases involved in gastric secretion.

   _____

   _____

   _____

   _____

©2008 Pearson Education, Inc.
Anatomy & Physiology for Emergency Care, 2nd ed.

17 Nutrition and Metabolism

Chapter Objectives

Content Self-Evaluation

MULTIPLE CHOICE

_____ 1. Which of the following best describes metabolism?
   A. the build up of organic material
   B. the breakdown of organic material
   C. all chemical reactions that occur in the body
   D. the absorption of nutrients

_____ 2. _____ is the synthesis of new organic molecules.
A. Catabolism C. Metabolism
B. Anabolism D. Nutrition

_____ 3. The process of breaking down large organic material to small organic molecules is called
_____.
A. metabolism C. catabolism
B. anabolism D. oxidation

_____ 4. All of the following are reasons for the synthesis of new organic compounds *except*
_____.
A. to build nutrient reserves C. to perform structural repairs
B. to support growth D. to decrease secretions

_____ 5. The most important product of metabolism is _____.
A. oxygen C. ATP
B. carbon dioxide D. glucose

_____ 6. Which of the following reactions represents the equation for normal carbohydrate
metabolism?
A. $C_6H_{12}O_6 + 6\ CO_2 \rightarrow 6\ O_2 + 6\ H_2O$ C. $C_6H_{12}O_6 + 6\ H_2O \rightarrow 6\ O_2 + 6\ CO_2$
B. $C_6H_{12}O_6 + 6\ O_2 \rightarrow 6\ CO_2 + 6\ H_2O$ D. $C_6H_{12}O_6 + 6\ O_2 \rightarrow 6\ O_2 + 6\ H_2O$

_____ 7. During the complete catabolism of one glucose molecule, a cell will gain _____ ATP
molecules.
A. 30 C. 34
B. 32 D. 36

_____ 8. During the process of glycolysis, glucose is broken into two 3-carbon molecules called
_____.
A. acetic acid C. citric acid
B. pyruvic acid D. acetyl-CoA

_____ 9. For the process of glycolysis to occur, all of the following are essential *except*
_____.
A. glucose C. oxygen
B. ATP and ADP D. NAD

_____ 10. During glycolysis, there is a net gain of _____ ATP molecules for each glucose
molecule converted.
A. 2 C. 36
B. 4 D. 38

_____ 11. Ninety-five percent of the ATP that is generated for cells to survive is made in
_____.
A. the citric acid cycle C. the TCA cycle
B. glycolysis D. the electron transport system

_____ 12. ATP is produced in which of the following organelles?
A. Golgi apparatus C. nucleus
B. lysosome D. mitochondria

_____ 13. The electron transport system is embedded within the _____.
A. outer mitochondrial membrane
B. inner mitochondrial membrane
C. inner membrane of the Golgi apparatus
D. outer membrane of the Golgi apparatus

_____ 14. In patients who are hypoxic, glycolysis continues to make an abundance of pyruvic acid,
which is converted into the dangerous _____.
A. citric acid C. lactic acid
B. carboxylic acid D. pyruvate

©2008 Pearson Education, Inc.
Anatomy & Physiology for Emergency Care, 2nd ed.

_____ 15. The synthesis of glucose from noncarbohydrate molecules is called _____.
    A. glycolysis
    B. glycogenolysis
    C. gluconeogenesis
    D. glycogenesis

_____ 16. _____ is an important energy reserve found in the liver and skeletal muscle.
    A. Glucose
    B. Glycogen
    C. Sucrose
    D. Fructose

_____ 17. The process of breaking down lipids into pieces that can be converted into pyruvic acid is called _____.
    A. lipogenesis
    B. lipolysis
    C. hydrolysis
    D. lipogenolysis

_____ 18. The catabolism of one fatty acid molecule generates _____ ATP molecules.
    A. 72
    B. 90
    C. 122
    D. 144

_____ 19. High-density lipoproteins are normally formed in the _____.
    A. small intestine
    B. large intestine
    C. liver
    D. pancreas

_____ 20. Which of the following types of lipoproteins is considered "bad cholesterol" and is most likely to contribute to arterial plaque?
    A. high-density lipoproteins
    B. triglycerides
    C. low-density lipoproteins
    D. free fatty acids

_____ 21. When an amino group from an amino acid is transferred to another carbon chain, which creates a new amino acid, this is called _____.
    A. deamination
    B. transamination
    C. urea formation
    D. ketosis

_____ 22. To eliminate toxic ammonia, the liver combines carbon dioxide with ammonia to form _____.
    A. ketone bodies
    B. amino acids
    C. urea
    D. ketosis

_____ 23. How many of the 22 amino acids are considered essential?
    A. 8
    B. 10
    C. 12
    D. 14

_____ 24. All of the following are examples of essential amino acids _except_ _____.
    A. alanine
    B. lysine
    C. phenylalanine
    D. valine

_____ 25. Which of the following types of diabetes typically requires insulin administration?
    A. Type I
    B. Type II
    C. Type III
    D. Type IV

_____ 26. You are evaluating a 56-year-old male who was found unconscious by a neighbor. The neighbor tells you that your patient is a diabetic. Your patient is breathing 45 times a minute. You notice the respirations to be deep and fast. You check his blood glucose level and it comes back at 350 mg/dL. (A normal level is 60–110 mg/dL.) What do you think is wrong with your patient?
    A. hypoglycemia
    B. diabetic ketoacidosis
    C. non-ketotic hyperosmolar coma
    D. hyperglycemia

_____ 27. Phenylketonuria is an inherited disease that prevents the conversion of the amino acid phenylalanine to the amino acid _____.
    A. valine
    B. leucine
    C. lysine
    D. tyrosine

_____ 28. An elevated uric acid level can lead to which of the following medical conditions?
A. renal stones
B. gall stones
C. gout
D. pancreatitis

_____ 29. All of the following are true regarding vitamins *except* _____.
A. vitamins are organic compounds
B. vitamins are required for normal metabolism and growth
C. vitamins are stored in the liver
D. vitamins are inorganic compounds

_____ 30. Which of the following vitamins is produced by the skin with exposure to the sun?
A. A
B. B
C. C
D. D

_____ 31. _____ is also called thiamine and is essential for carbohydrate metabolism.
A. B_1
B. B_2
C. B_6
D. B_{12}

_____ 32. In developing countries, the disease beriberi is caused by a deficiency in _____.
A. vitamin K
B. vitamin B_{12}
C. vitamin D
D. vitamin B_1

_____ 33. Which of the following food categories should be used sparingly?
A. grains
B. vegetables
C. fats
D. meat and beans

_____ 34. _____ is the result of conductive heat loss into the air that overlies the surface of an object.
A. Radiation
B. Conduction
C. Convection
D. Evaporation

_____ 35. Which of the following mechanisms of heat transfer is the direct transfer of energy through physical contact?
A. radiation
B. conduction
C. convection
D. evaporation

_____ 36. An average individual has a basal metabolic rate of _____ calories per hour or about _____ calories per day.
A. 100, 2400
B. 60, 1440
C. 70, 1680
D. 80, 1920

_____ 37. The heat-loss centers in the central nervous system are in the _____.
A. cerebrum
B. cerebellum
C. thalamus
D. hypothalamus

_____ 38. All of the following are ways to promote heat loss *except* _____.
A. sweating
B. vasodilation
C. vasoconstriction
D. increase in respirations

_____ 39. All of the following are reasons for fire-ground personnel to report to the rehabilitation area *except* _____.
A. strenuous activity, including forced entry
B. failure of an SCBA unit
C. 30 minutes of operation within a hazardous materials area
D. the use and depletion of one self-contained breathing apparatus (SCBA)

_____ 40. Good nutrition is important for all EMS personnel. Which of the following is considered a healthy breakdown of the types and quantities of food that should be eaten each day?
A. 30 percent carbohydrates, 60 percent protein, 10 percent fat
B. 40 percent carbohydrates, 40 percent protein, 20 percent fat
C. 60 percent carbohydrates, 30 percent protein, 10 percent fat
D. 40 percent carbohydrates, 20 percent protein, 40 percent fat

_____ 41. Foods that are low in dietary fiber are _____.
     A. rice and pasta   C. fruits
     B. cereals   D. meats

_____ 42. The breakdown of lipids generates approximately _____ calories per gram of energy.
     A. 4   C. 9
     B. 6   D. 12

_____ 43. The breakdown of carbohydrates generates approximately_____ calories per gram of energy.
     A. 2   C. 9
     B. 4   D. 12

_____ 44. An individual's basal metabolic rate can be affected by _____.
     A. gender   C. genetics
     B. age   D. All of the above.

_____ 45. In the average geriatric patient, changes in health and food intake are related to _____.
     A. lifestyle changes   C. a change in eating habits
     B. income   D. All of the above.

FILL IN THE BLANK

1. Carbohydrates are considered the first source of energy. The breakdown of _____ is second.

2. _____ are organic molecules, usually derived from vitamins, that must be present for an enzymatic reaction to occur.

3. To produce 36 ATP from glucose, the body also needs to have _____ available.

4. Another term for aerobic metabolism is _____.

5. _____ is the coenzyme that is responsible for the removal of the hydrogen atoms during glycolysis.

6. The process of adding a phosphate group to ADP to form ATP is called _____.

7. The enzyme that is responsible for allowing hydrogen ions to diffuse back into the mitochondrial matrix through a membrane is called _____.

8. The carbons found within the glucose molecule are converted into _____.

9. The synthesis of lipids is known as _____.

10. Because HDL does not cause circulatory problems, it is called _____.

11. In amino acid catabolism, the removal of the amino group from the amino acid requires a coenzyme derived from _____.

12. The largest of all lipoproteins are called _____.

13. _____ is the process that prepares an amino acid for breakdown in the tricarboxylic acid cycle (TCA).

14. Organic acids that are produced during lipid catabolism are called _____.

15. The increase in the production of ketone bodies that occurs during protein and lipid catabolism causes a condition called _____.

16. A condition in which there is an excess amount of available glucose is called _____.

17. Individuals of any age with a total cholesterol of less than _____ have a low cholesterol level and are at low risk for heart disease.

18. _____ are inorganic molecules released through the dissociation of electrolytes.

19. The two primary nervous system diseases that are caused by thiamine deficiencies are _____ and _____.

20. More than half of the heat we lose through our skin is through _____.

MATCHING

Match the terms in Column A with the words or phrases in Column B. Write the letter of the corresponding words or phrases in the spaces provided.

Column A

_____ 1. pyrexia

_____ 2. hypothermia

_____ 3. ketonuria

_____ 4. heat exhaustion

_____ 5. ketosis

_____ 6. glycolysis

_____ 7. lipolysis

_____ 8. deamination

_____ 9. heat stroke

_____ 10. glycogen

Column B

a. malfunction of the thermoregulatory system

b. lipid catabolism

c. removal of amino group

d. a condition in which the thermoregulatory center stops functioning and body temperature rises uncontrollably

e. elevated body temperature

f. large glucose molecule

g. below normal body temperature

h. ketones in the urine

i. high concentration of ketone bodies

j. breakdown of glucose to pyruvic acid

©2008 Pearson Education, Inc.
Anatomy & Physiology for Emergency Care, 2nd ed.

LABELING EXERCISE 17–1

Identify the elements in the TCA cycle shown in Figure 17–1. Place the corresponding letter on the line next to the appropriate label. Please use each letter only once.

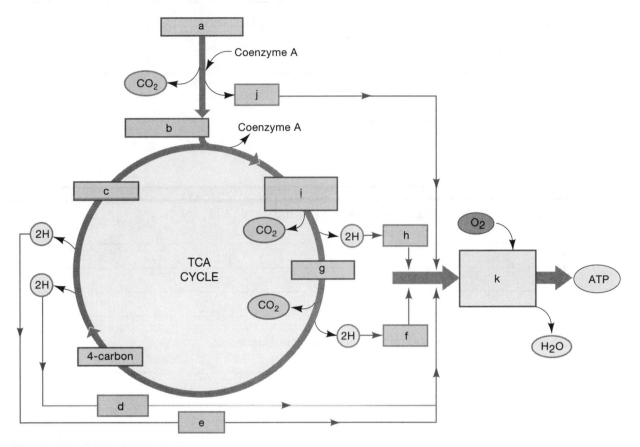

Figure 17–1 The TCA Cycle

_____ 1. NADH

_____ 2. pyruvic acid

_____ 3. 5-carbon

_____ 4. acetyl CoA

_____ 5. NADH

_____ 6. 4-carbon

_____ 7. citric acid 6-carbon

_____ 8. FADH$_2$

_____ 9. NADH

_____ 10. NADH

_____ 11. electron transport system

SHORT ANSWER

1. Discuss the differences between glycolysis and the tricarboxylic acid (TCA) cycle.

_____

_____

_____

_____

_____

_____

2. Define the term cellular respiration.

_____

3. Discuss the impact of cellular hypoxia on the production of ATP.

_____

_____

_____

_____

4. Discuss the differences between deamination and transamination.

_____

_____

_____

_____

5. Discuss the differences between hypoglycemia and hyperglycemia.

_____

_____

_____

©2008 Pearson Education, Inc.
Anatomy & Physiology for Emergency Care, 2nd ed.

18 The Urinary System

Chapter Objectives

Content Self-Evaluation

MULTIPLE CHOICE

_____ 1. All of the following are functions of the urinary system *except* _____.
A. regulating blood pressure through the release of renin
B. stabilizing blood pH
C. regulating plasma concentrations of ions
D. All of the above are functions of the urinary system.

_____ 2. The indentation where the ureter leaves the kidney is called the _____.
A. renal cortex
B. hilum
C. renal medulla
D. renal pyramid

_____ 3. Which of the following body systems are responsible for coordinating metabolic activities with the urinary system?
A. nervous, lymphatic, and cardiovascular
B. digestive, respiratory, and cardiovascular
C. muscular, endocrine, and digestive
D. nervous, digestive, and endocrine

_____ 4. The kidney is divided into sections called the _____.
A. minor and major calyces
B. nephrons and capillaries
C. cortex and medulla
D. papilla and pyramids

_____ 5. As the renal arteries enter the renal sinuses, they branch into the _____ arteries.
A. interlobar
B. acuate
C. interlobular
D. vasa recta

_____ 6. Blood arrives at the glomerulus by way of the _____.
A. efferent arteriole
B. afferent arteriole
C. peritubular capillaries
D. vasa recta

_____ 7. The basic functioning unit of the kidney is the _____.
A. distal convoluted tubule
B. proximal convoluted tubule
C. loop of Henle
D. nephron

_____ 8. The kidneys are held in position in the retroperitoneal space by the _____.
A. major calyx, minor calyx, and renal medulla
B. overlying peritoneum, supporting connective tissues, and contact with other organs
C. renal pyramids, renal sinus, and renal corpuscle
D. major calyx, minor calyx, and renal pyramids

_____ 9. In the juxtamedullary nephrons, the peritubular capillaries are directly connected to the _____.
A. arcuate arteries
B. vasa recta
C. renal arteries
D. cortical nephrons

_____ 10. The production of urine occurs in the _____.
A. bladder
B. urethra
C. ureter
D. kidney

_____ 11. The renal corpuscle consists of the _____.
A. proximal and distal convoluted tubules
B. glomerulus and Bowman's capsule
C. renal pyramids
D. loop of Henle

_____ 12. Podocytes are specialized filtration cells found in the _____.
A. vasa recta
B. ascending loop of Henle
C. bladder
D. glomerulus

_____ 13. Which of the following lists the regions of the nephron in the correct order of flow?
    A. distal convoluted tubule, loop of Henle, proximal convoluted tubule, glomerular capsule
    B. proximal convoluted tubule, loop of Henle, distal convoluted tubule, glomerular capsule
    C. glomerular capsule, proximal convoluted tubule, loop of Henle, distal convoluted tubule
    D. loop of Henle, proximal convoluted tubule, distal convoluted tubule, glomerular capsule

_____ 14. Which of the following is the correct order of blood flow through the kidneys?
    A. efferent arteriole, afferent arteriole, glomerulus, peritubular capillaries
    B. afferent arterioles, glomerulus, efferent arterioles, peritubular capillaries
    C. afferent arterioles, glomerulus, peritubular capillaries, efferent arterioles
    D. efferent arterioles, glomerulus, afferent arterioles, peritubular capillaries

_____ 15. The ascending loop of Henle is responsible for _____.
    A. the reabsorption of water
    B. the reabsorption and transport of sodium and chloride ions
    C. the movement of urine into the minor calyx
    D. the reabsorption of calcium

_____ 16. Which of the following components of the nephron has the greatest impact on controlling the blood pressure?
    A. afferent arteriole   C. peritubular capillaries
    B. efferent arteriole   D. loop of Henle

_____ 17. The proximal and distal convoluted tubules are comprised of what type of epithelial cells?
    A. simple squamous   C. transitional
    B. simple cuboidal   D. stratified squamous

_____ 18. The solute found in the glomerular capsule must be small enough to pass through all of the following portions of the capsule *except* _____.
    A. the pores of the endothelial cells
    B. the fibers of the basement membrane
    C. the filtration slits of the capillary
    D. the pores found within the epithelial cells

_____ 19. Which of the following two components of the renal system comprise the juxtaglomerular apparatus?
    A. distal convoluted tubules, loop of Henle
    B. juxtaglomerular cells, macula densa
    C. macula densa, distal convoluted tubule
    D. juxtaglomerular cells, loop of Henle

_____ 20. The juxtaglomerular apparatus is the endocrine structure that secretes _____.
    A. renin and angiotensin I   C. ADH and renin
    B. angiotensin I and erythropoietin   D. renin and erythropoietin

_____ 21. The last segment of the nephron that opens into the collecting system is the _____.
    A. loop of Henle   C. proximal convoluted tubule
    B. distal convoluted tubule   D. glomerulus

_____ 22. The most abundant organic waste found in urine is _____.
    A. creatinine   C. urea
    B. uric acid   D. lactic acid

_____ 23. All of the following are metabolic waste products found in urine *except* _____.
    A. urea   C. proteins
    B. uric acid   D. creatinine

_____ 24. The glomerular filtration rate (GFR) refers to _____.
   A. the amount of filtrate produced in the kidneys each minute
   B. the amount of filtrate produced in the kidneys each second
   C. the amount of filtrate produced in the kidneys each hour
   D. the amount of filtrate produced in the kidneys each day

_____ 25. In the course of a single day, the glomeruli produce _____ of filtrate.
   A. 100 liters   C. 150 liters
   B. 120 liters   D. 180 liters

_____ 26. The proximal convoluted tubule is known to reabsorb all of the following *except* _____.
   A. sodium   C. potassium
   B. hydrogen ions   D. glucose

_____ 27. Which of the following segments of the nephron is impermeable to both water and solutes?
   A. proximal convoluted tubule   C. ascending limb of loop of Henle
   B. distal convoluted tubule   D. descending limb of loop of Henle

_____ 28. Ion pumps that respond to the hormone aldosterone are located in the _____.
   A. distal convoluted tubule   C. glomerulus
   B. proximal convoluted tubule D. loop of Henle

_____ 29. Circulating levels of _____ control the reabsorption of water along the distal convoluted tubule and collecting ducts.
   A. renin   C. angiotensin II
   B. antidiuretic hormone   D. angiotensin I

_____ 30. Which of the following substances is normally completely reabsorbed by the tubules of the nephron?
   A. creatinine   C. sodium
   B. glucose   D. uric acid

_____ 31. If the level of aldosterone is increased in the blood, the _____.
   A. sodium levels decrease D. blood pressure decreases
   B. sodium levels increase E. both B and C
   C. blood pressure elevates F. both A and D

_____ 32. All of the following are ways the glomerular filtration rate is controlled *except* _____.
   A. local automatic adjustments in glomerular pressures
   B. the sympathetic nervous system
   C. the parasympathetic nervous system
   D. various hormones

_____ 33. The normal daily volume of urine produced is _____.
   A. 200 to 400 mL   C. 1000 to 1200 mL
   B. 400 to 600 mL   D. 1500 to 2000 mL

_____ 34. The renin that is released from the juxtaglomerular apparatus converts _____ to help regulate blood pressure.
   A. angiotensin I to angiotensin II   C. angiotensinogen to angiotensin I
   B. angiotensinogen to angiotensin II   D. angiotensin II to angiotensin I

_____ 35. An angiotensin-converting enzyme is responsible for converting _____.
   A. angiotensinogen to angiotensin I   C. angiotensin I to angiotensin II
   B. angiotensinogen to angiotensin II   D. angiotensin II to angiotensin I

©2008 Pearson Education, Inc.
Anatomy & Physiology for Emergency Care, 2nd ed.

_____ 36. If an elevated pressure in the atrial wall of the heart is recognized by the atrial natriuretic peptides, this causes all of the following to occur *except* _____.
   A. a decrease in the rate of sodium reabsorption in the distal convoluted tubules
   B. dilation of the glomerular capillaries
   C. inactivation of the renin-angiotensin system
   D. an increase in renin release from the juxtaglomerular apparatus

_____ 37. The most common ion that causes kidney stones (renal calculi) is _____.
   A. magnesium
   B. sodium
   C. calcium
   D. chloride

_____ 38. The tissue that makes up most of the bladder is _____.
   A. simple cuboidal epithelium
   B. simple columnar epithelium
   C. transitional epithelium
   D. squamous epithelium

_____ 39. The triangular area of the bladder that forms the entrance into the urethra is called the _____.
   A. detrusor
   B. trigone
   C. symphysis
   D. ureter

_____ 40. The primary micturition reflex in the bladder is controlled by the _____.
   A. sympathetic nervous system
   B. cerebellum
   C. parasympathetic nervous system
   D. thalamus

_____ 41. Contraction of the muscular bladder forces the urine out of the body through the _____.
   A. ureter
   B. urethra
   C. bladder
   D. All of the above.

_____ 42. The principle cation found in the intracellular fluid is _____.
   A. potassium
   B. calcium
   C. sodium
   D. magnesium

_____ 43. Intracellular fluid can be found _____.
   A. inside blood vessels
   B. in the interstitial spaces
   C. inside the cell
   D. in the cerebrospinal fluid

_____ 44. The principle cation found within the extracellular fluid is _____.
   A. potassium
   B. calcium
   C. sodium
   D. magnesium

_____ 45. Cardiac arrhythmias may occur if the extracellular concentrations of _____ become too high.
   A. sodium
   B. potassium
   C. magnesium
   D. chloride

_____ 46. If the extracellular fluid becomes more concentrated with respect to the intracellular fluid, water will move _____.
   A. from the extracellular fluid to inside the cells
   B. against the gradient using active transport
   C. from the cell to the extracellular fluid
   D. No fluid will move because the two areas are equal.

_____ 47. If the intracellular fluid becomes more concentrated with respect to the extracellular fluid, water will move _____.
   A. from the extracellular fluid into the cells
   B. against the gradient using active transport
   C. from the cell to the extracellular fluid
   D. No fluid will move because the two areas are equal.

_____ 48. An increase in carbon dioxide levels in the blood causes the pH to _____.
   A. increase
   B. stay the same
   C. drop

_____ 49. An increase in carbon dioxide levels in the blood will cause a patient's breathing rate to _____.
   A. increase   C. decrease slightly
   B. decrease   D. stay the same

_____ 50. The normal range for the pH of the blood is _____.
   A. 7.00 to 7.35   C. 7.45 to 7.55
   B. 7.35 to 7.45   D. 7.25 to 7.35

_____ 51. When the pH of the blood is below 7.35, this is called _____.
   A. normal   C. acidosis
   B. alkalosis   D. None of the above.

_____ 52. Hypernatremia is a condition characterized by elevations of _____ in the blood.
   A. sodium   C. calcium
   B. potassium   D. magnesium

_____ 53. Which of the following acid-base imbalances is caused from prolonged vomiting?
   A. respiratory acidosis   C. metabolic acidosis
   B. respiratory alkalosis   D. metabolic alkalosis

_____ 54. Chronic obstructive pulmonary disease is a respiratory disease that may cause which of the following acid-base imbalances?
   A. respiratory acidosis   C. metabolic acidosis
   B. respiratory alkalosis   D. metabolic alkalosis

_____ 55. Urination in the elderly occurs more frequently due to _____.
   A. a decrease in ADH
   B. incontinence
   C. an increase in ADH production
   D. nephrons not recognizing or responding to the ADH

Fill in the Blank

1. Most of the organic waste in the blood is removed by the _____.

2. The primary purpose of _____ production is to maintain homeostasis by regulating the volume and composition of the blood.

3. Urine production occurs in the renal _____.

4. Blood reaches each nephron initially through the _____.

5. _____ is produced during the breakdown and recycling of RNA.

6. The epithelium that covers the glomerular capillaries consists of cells called _____.

7. _____ is the inability to control urination voluntarily.

8. _____ is a metabolic waste product excreted by the kidneys that plays a role in muscle contraction.

9. The proximal convoluted tubule reclaims _____ percent of the filtrate produced at the glomerulus.

10. The distal convoluted tubule and collecting ducts contain ion pumps that respond to the hormone _____ which is produced by the adrenal cortex.

©2008 Pearson Education, Inc.
Anatomy & Physiology for Emergency Care, 2nd ed.

11. Autonomic regulation of kidney function is controlled primarily by the _____ branch of the autonomic nervous system.

12. _____ is due to a decrease in alveolar ventilation, which results in carbon dioxide retention.

13. The actions of the atrial natriuretic peptide (ANP) oppose the effects of the _____ system.

14. The _____ are muscular tubes that conduct urine from the kidneys to the urinary bladder.

15. Nephrolithiasis is the medical term for a _____.

ORDERING EXERCISE

Place the following steps of the reabsorption of water and the production of urine in the correct order using the letters A–F.

_____ 1. In the proximal convoluted tubule and descending loop of Henle, water moves into the surrounding interstitial fluid and leaves a small fluid volume of highly concentrated fluid.

_____ 2. The final composition and concentration of the tubular fluid are determined by activity in the descending convoluted tubule and the collecting ducts. These segments are impermeable to solutes, and only sodium ions can be transported in and out of the tubule due to the influence of aldosterone.

_____ 3. The concentration of urine is controlled by variations in the water permeability of the distal convoluted tubule and the collecting ducts. These segments are impermeable to water unless exposed to antidiuretic hormone (ADH).

_____ 4. Glomerular filtration produces a filtrate that resembles blood plasma. This filtrate has the same osmotic concentration as plasma.

_____ 5. The ascending limb of the loop of Henle is impermeable to water and solutes. The tubular cells actively pump sodium and chloride ions out of the tubular fluid.

_____ 6. In the proximal convoluted tubule, 60 to 70 percent of the water and almost all of the dissolved nutrients are reabsorbed.

MATCHING

Match the terms in Column A with the words or phrases in Column B. Write the letter of the corresponding words or phrases in the spaces provided.

Column A

_____ 1. juxtaglomerular apparatus

_____ 2. loop of Henle

_____ 3. distal convoluted tubule

_____ 4. proximal convoluted tubule

_____ 5. collecting ducts

_____ 6. renal cortex

_____ 7. renal medulla

_____ 8. renal pelvis

_____ 9. pyelonephritis

_____ 10. aldosterone

Column B

a. reabsorption of nutrients occurs here

b. urine production begins here

c. contains renal pyramids

d. associated with renin

e. regulation of sodium and water in the urine

f. continuous with the ureter

g. secreted by adrenal cortex

h. active site for the secretion of ions and drugs

i. inflammation of kidney tissue

j. respond to the hormone aldosterone

LABELING EXERCISE 18–1

Identify the structures of the kidney shown in Figure 18–1. Place the corresponding letter on the line next to the appropriate label.

_____ 1. Renal columns

_____ 2. Medulla

_____ 3. Renal pelvis

_____ 4. Major calyx

_____ 5. Renal papilla

_____ 6. Renal pyramids

_____ 7. Ureter

_____ 8. Cortex

_____ 9. Minor calyx

_____ 10. Renal sinus

_____ 11. Renal capsule

_____ 12. Hilum

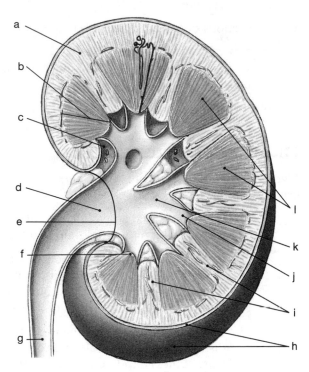

Figure 18–1 The Structure of the Kidney

LABELING EXERCISE 18–2

Identify the parts of the juxtamedullary nephron shown in Figure 18–2. Place the corresponding letter on the line next to the appropriate label.

_____ 1. Afferent arteriole

_____ 2. Vasa recta

_____ 3. Proximal convoluted tubule

_____ 4. Loop of Henle

_____ 5. Efferent arteriole

_____ 6. Glomerulus

_____ 7. Peritubular capillaries

_____ 8. Distal convoluted tubule

_____ 9. Collecting duct

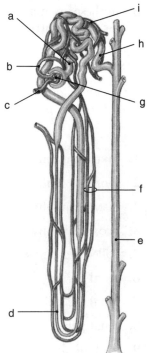

Figure 18–2 A Juxtamedullary Nephron

©2008 Pearson Education, Inc.
Anatomy & Physiology for Emergency Care, 2nd ed.

LABELING EXERCISE 18–3

Identify the structures of the nephron and collecting system shown in Figure 18–3. Place the corresponding letter on the line next to the appropriate label.

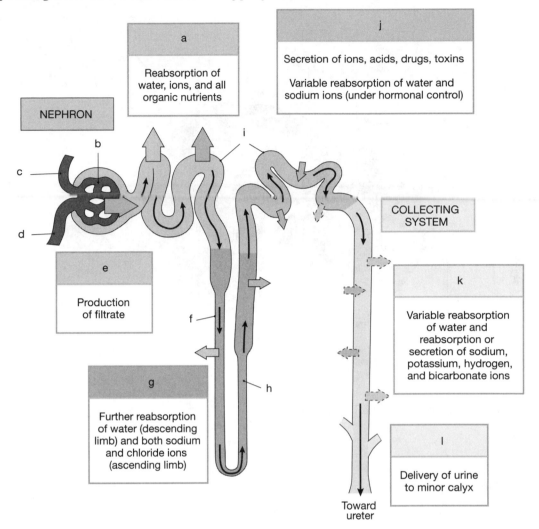

Figure 18–3 A Nephron and the Collecting System

_____ 1. Glomerulus

_____ 2. Collecting duct

_____ 3. Ascending limb

_____ 4. Proximal convoluted tubule

_____ 5. Afferent arteriole

_____ 6. Loop of Henle

_____ 7. Renal corpuscle

_____ 8. Distal convoluted tubule

_____ 9. Efferent arteriole

_____ 10. Papillary duct

_____ 11. Descending limb

_____ 12. Renal tubule

LABELING EXERCISE 18–4

Identify the structural features of the renal corpuscle shown in Figure 18–4. Place the corresponding letter on the line next to the appropriate label.

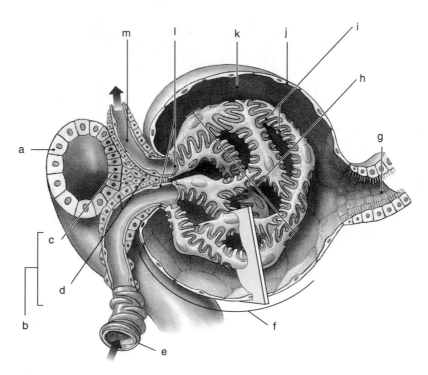

Figure 18–4 The Renal Corpuscle

_____ 1. Macula densa

_____ 2. Podocyte processes (pedicels)

_____ 3. Afferent arteriole

_____ 4. Glomerular capillary

_____ 5. Distal convoluted tubule

_____ 6. Efferent arteriole

_____ 7. Proximal convoluted tubule

_____ 8. Juxtaglomerular cells

_____ 9. Capsular space

_____ 10. Capsular epithelium

_____ 11. Juxtaglomerular apparatus

_____ 12. Glomerulus

_____ 13. Bowman's capsule

LABELING EXERCISE 18–5

Identify the parts of the male urinary bladder shown in Figure 18–5. Place the corresponding letter on the line next to the appropriate label.

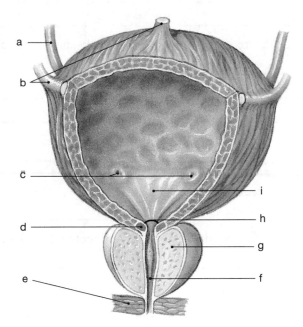

Figure 18–5 The Male Urinary Bladder

_____ 1. Ligaments

_____ 2. External urethral sphincter

_____ 3. Prostate gland

_____ 4. Trigone

_____ 5. Ureteral openings

_____ 6. Internal urethral sphincter

_____ 7. Urethra

_____ 8. Neck

_____ 9. Ureter

SHORT ANSWER

1. Discuss the role of hemodialysis in the field of medicine today.

   _____

   _____

   _____

2. Describe the role of atrial natriuretic peptide (ANP) in fluid balance in the body.

   _____

   _____

   _____

3. Describe the signs and symptoms typically seen with kidney stones.

   _____

   _____

   _____

4. Discuss the differences between metabolic acidosis and metabolic alkalosis.

   _____

   _____

   _____

   _____

5. List the five age-related changes that occur to the urinary system in the elderly.

   _____

   _____

   _____

   _____

   _____

19 The Reproductive System

Chapter Objectives

Content Self-Evaluation

MULTIPLE CHOICE

_____ 1. Upon fertilization of the egg, a single cell is created and is called the _____.
   A. gamete
   B. gonad
   C. zygote
   D. ova

_____ 2. All of the following comprise the male reproductive tract *except* the _____.
   A. epididymis
   B. ejaculatory duct
   C. ductus deferens
   D. prostate gland

_____ 3. Which of the following muscles is responsible for pulling the testes closer to the body?
   A. dartos
   B. scrotal
   C. cremaster
   D. urethra

_____ 4. Normal sperm development requires the scrotal temperature to be _____ that of the body.
  A. higher than   C. lower than
  B. the same as   D. Sperm will develop at any temperature.

_____ 5. The dense fibrous capsule that surrounds the testicle is called the _____.
  A. seminiferous tubule   C. tunica albuginea
  B. prostate   D. sustentacular cells

_____ 6. The sustentacular cells are responsible for _____.
  A. producing testosterone   C. producing semen
  B. nourishing the developing sperm cells   D. producing androgens

_____ 7. A special form of cell division that produces gametes is called _____.
  A. mitosis   C. spermatagonia
  B. meiosis   D. spermiogenesis

_____ 8. During mitosis the immature sperm cells are called _____.
  A. spermatids   C. spermatogonia
  B. spermatozoa   D. secondary spermocytes

_____ 9. Spermatogenesis is the process that produces _____.
  A. spermatids   C. spermatozoa
  B. secondary spermatocytes   D. spermatogonia

_____ 10. At the end of meiosis, spermatocytes produce immature gametes called _____.
  A. spermatids   C. spermatogonia
  B. secondary spermatocytes   D. spermatozoa

_____ 11. The exchange called _____ increases genetic variation among offspring.
  A. synapsis   C. tetrad
  B. crossing over   D. metaphase

_____ 12. Enzymes found in the sperm that are essential for fertilization are located in the _____.
  A. head of the sperm   C. acrosomal cap
  B. neck   D. tail

_____ 13. The tail of the sperm is the only example of a _____ found in the human body.
  A. lysosome   C. peroxisome
  B. flagellum   D. endoplasmic reticulum

_____ 14. The functions of the epididymis include all of the following *except* _____.
  A. adjust the fluid composition from the seminiferous tubules
  B. recycle damaged spermatozoa
  C. store maturing spermatozoa
  D. produce semen

_____ 15. Which of the following is the correct route sperm would take to exit the body?
  A. epididymis, ejaculatory duct, ductus deferens, urethra
  B. epididymis, ductus deferens, ejaculatory duct, urethra
  C. ductus deferens, epididymis, urethra, ejaculatory duct
  D. ejaculatory duct, epididymis, urethra, ductus deferens

_____ 16. Sperm production occurs within the _____.
  A. prostate gland   C. seminiferous tubules
  B. epididymis   D. ductus deferens

_____ 17. The junction of the ductus deferens and the _____ comprise the structure known as the ejaculatory duct.
  A. prostate gland   C. testes
  B. seminal vesicle   D. Bartholin's gland

©2008 Pearson Education, Inc.
Anatomy & Physiology for Emergency Care, 2nd ed.

_____ 18. The accessory organs that are responsible for secreting the majority of the seminal fluid are the _____.
A. epididymis, ductus deferens, and prostate gland
B. prostate gland, seminal vesicle, and bulbourethral glands
C. adrenal gland, ductus deferens, and epididymis
D. prostate gland, epididymis, and seminal vesicle

_____ 19. All of the following are functions of the accessory glands *except* _____.
A. activating the spermatozoa
B. providing nutrients for the spermatozoa
C. generating peristaltic contractions to propel the spermatozoa
D. producing an acidic environment to counteract the alkaline vaginal environment

_____ 20. Semen contained in the seminal vesicle provides all of the following for the sperm *except* _____.
A. fructose for energy
B. prostaglandins to help stimulate smooth muscle contraction
C. fibrinogen
D. plasminogen

_____ 21. The _____ found at the base of the penis produce(s) a lubricating secretion.
A. Bartholin's gland
B. prostate gland
C. seminal vesicle
D. bulbourethral glands

_____ 22. The gland that surrounds the urethra as it leaves the urinary bladder and produces an acidic solution is called the _____.
A. bulbourethral gland
B. seminal vesicle
C. prostate gland
D. Bartholin's gland

_____ 23. The gland that provides 60 percent of the volume of semen is called the _____.
A. seminal vesicle
B. bulbourethral gland
C. Bartholin's gland
D. prostate gland

_____ 24. Within the prostatic fluid is a substance called seminalplasmin that is responsible for _____.
A. providing the alkaline solution for the semen
B. providing the fructose necessary for the sperm to survive
C. serving as an antibiotic that reduces urinary tract infections in men
D. providing fibrinogen that stimulates clotting within the vagina

_____ 25. In patients who have received a high spinal cord injury, priapism may occur due to _____.
A. unopposed sympathetic stimulation
B. stimulation of the twelfth cranial nerve
C. unopposed parasympathetic stimulation
D. stimulation of the eighth cranial nerve

_____ 26. The hormone that is synthesized by the hypothalamus and carried to the anterior pituitary gland is called _____.
A. gonadotropin-releasing hormone (GnRH)
B. follicle-stimulating hormone (FSH)
C. luteinizing hormone (LH)
D. interstitial cell-stimulating hormone (ICSH)

_____ 27. Which of the following hormones is responsible for stimulating spermatogenesis?
A. LH
B. FSH
C. ICSH
D. GnRH

_____ 28. _____ is the hormone that is responsible for the secretion of testosterone in males.
A. FSH
B. ADH
C. LH
D. TSH

_____ 29. The _____ are (is) responsible for the production of female gametes and the secretion of female sex hormones.
A. uterus
C. endometrium
B. myometrium
D. ovaries

_____ 30. At which of the following ages do the primary oocytes begin meiosis?
A. three to seven months of age
C. five to seven years of age
B. from birth to one year of age
D. eleven to twelve years of age

_____ 31. The signal to complete meiosis occurs when the female _____.
A. becomes an adult
C. is born
B. reaches puberty
D. completes first uterine cycle

_____ 32. During the process of oogenesis, three non-functioning polar bodies are formed along with a(n) _____.
A. primordial follicle
C. antrum
B. ovum
D. zona pellucida

_____ 33. A normal ovarian cycle lasts for _____ days.
A. 7
C. 21
B. 14
D. 28

_____ 34. The muscular layer of the uterus is called the _____.
A. endometrium
C. perimetrium
B. myometrium
D. epimetrium

_____ 35. The first uterine cycle is also called _____.
A. menses
C. menarche
B. the menstrual cycle
D. menopause

_____ 36. Pelvic pain with the onset of menses is called _____.
A. dyspareunia
C. dysmenorrhea
B. dyspnea
D. amenorrhea

_____ 37. Which of the following phases occurs within days of the completion of the menstrual cycle?
A. secretory phase
C. luteal phase
B. ovarian phase
D. proliferative phase

_____ 38. Which of the following phases occurs when the endometrium prepares for the arrival of the developing embryo?
A. secretory phase
C. follicular phase
B. proliferative phase
D. ovarian phase

_____ 39. During menstruation _____.
A. a new uterine lining is formed
B. ovulation occurs
C. the old endometrial layer is sloughed off
D. the corpus luteum is formed

_____ 40. The erectile tissue that is located just anterior to the vaginal opening is called the _____.
A. perineum
C. clitoris
B. vulva
D. labia minora

_____ 41. Which of the following hormones causes the final development of the breasts into milk-secreting glands?
A. estrogen
C. progesterone
B. prolactin
D. oxytocin

_____ 42. Which of the following is _not_ a risk factor for breast cancer in women?
A. family history of breast cancer
C. early menarche
B. first pregnancy after the age of 30
D. early menopause

_____ 43. All of the following are functions of estrogen *except* _____.
  A. stimulating bone and muscle growth
  B. maintaining secondary sex characteristics
  C. maintaining accessory reproductive glands
  D. All of the above are functions of estrogen.

_____ 44. Which of the following hormones triggers ovulation?
  A. luteinizing hormone   C. gonadotropin-releasing hormone
  B. follicle-stimulating hormone D. inhibin

_____ 45. Menopause typically occurs between the ages of _____.
  A. 30 and 40   C. 45 and 55
  B. 40 and 45   D. 55 and 60

_____ 46. During menopause, there is a decline in the circulating concentrations of _____.
  A. GnRH   C. LH
  B. FSH   D. estrogen

_____ 47. At the point of puberty for males and females _____.
  A. levels of FSH and LH increase   C. oogenesis is accelerated in females
  B. secondary sex characteristics appear D. All of the above.

_____ 48. During arousal, stimulation of sensory nerves in the genital region increase the
          parasympathetic nervous system, which causes a(n) _____.
  A. emission   C. ejaculation
  B. erection   D. impotence

_____ 49. In males between the ages of 50 and 60, circulating levels of _____ decrease, while
          _____ levels increase.
  A. LH, FSH   C. FSH and LH, testosterone
  B. FSH, LH   D. testosterone, LH and FSH

_____ 50. The reported failure rate of condoms in preventing pregnancy is between _____.
  A. 3 and 5 percent   C. 6 and 17 percent
  B. 8 and 12 percent   D. 15 and 20 percent

FILL IN THE BLANK

1. The primary sex organs of the male are the _____.

2. In _____ one or both of the testes have failed to descend from the abdomen.

3. _____ occurs when the testicle twists on the spermatic cord.

4. _____ is part of the process of somatic cell division.

5. A matched set of four chromatids is called a _____.

6. During meiosis II the cells go from diploid to _____.

7. For sperm to become motile, they must undergo _____.

8. The fold of skin that covers the tip of the penis is called the _____.

9. Luteinizing hormone was once called _____ in males.

10. _____ is the medical definition for midcycle abdominal pain brought on by ovulation.

11. _____ is the medical definition for pain during sexual intercourse.

12. The end of the uterine tube that is closest to the ovary forms an expanded funnel or _____.

13. The disintegration of the _____ marks the end of the ovarian cycle.

14. The inferior portion of the uterus that projects into the vagina is called the _____.

15. The epithelial layer of the uterine wall contains _____ cells that are responsible for completing the capacitation of the spermatozoa.

16. _____ is a condition in which endometrial tissue is found outside of the uterus.

17. The most common cause of nontraumatic gynecological pain is _____.

18. The most common causes of pelvic inflammatory disease (PID) are _____ and _____.

19. The outer limits of the _____ are formed by the mons pubis and labia majora.

20. _____ is defined as an inability to achieve pregnancy after one year of appropriately timed sexual intercourse.

MATCHING

Match the terms in Column A with the words or phrases in Column B. Write the letter of the corresponding words or phrases in the spaces provided.

Column A

_____ 1. cervical cancer

_____ 2. vasectomy

_____ 3. orchitis

_____ 4. gynecology

_____ 5. mastectomy

_____ 6. prostatectomy

_____ 7. oophoritis

_____ 8. mammography

_____ 9. pelvic inflammatory disease

_____ 10. amenorrhea

Column B

a. study of the female reproductive tract

b. surgical removal of a cancerous mammary gland

c. inflammation of an ovary

d. X-ray used to examine breast tissue

e. the most common reproductive cancer in women

f. surgical removal of a segment of ductus deferens

g. infection of the uterine tube

h. inflammation of the testes

i. cessation of menstruation for 6 months or more

j. surgical removal of prostate gland

LABELING EXERCISE 19–1

Identify the parts of the male reproductive system shown in Figure 19–1. Place the corresponding letter on the line next to the appropriate label.

_____ 1. Penis

_____ 2. Ejaculatory duct

_____ 3. Prepuce

_____ 4. Seminal vesicle

_____ 5. Epididymis

_____ 6. Glans

_____ 7. Ureter

_____ 8. Ductus deferens

_____ 9. Pubic symphysis

_____ 10. Scrotum

_____ 11. Prostate gland

_____ 12. Urethra

_____ 13. Bulbourethral gland

_____ 14. Testis

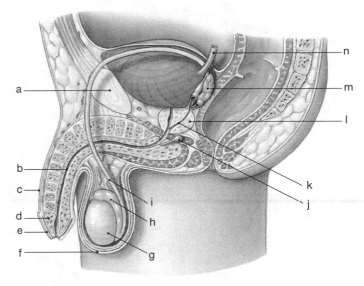

Figure 19–1 The Male Reproductive System

LABELING EXERCISE 19–2

Identify the reproductive structures shown in Figure 19–2. Place the corresponding letter on the line next to the appropriate label.

_____ 1. Ductus deferens

_____ 2. Prostate gland

_____ 3. Seminal vesicle

_____ 4. Ejaculatory duct

_____ 5. Ureter

_____ 6. Urethra

_____ 7. Bulbourethral gland

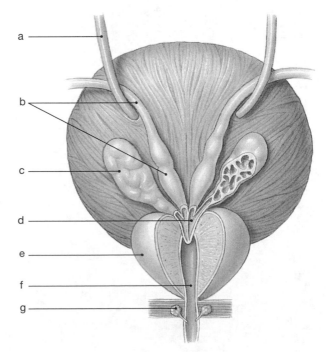

Figure 19–2 Reproductive Structures

LABELING EXERCISE 19–3

Identify the parts of the female reproductive system shown in Figure 19–3. Place the corresponding letter on the line next to the appropriate label.

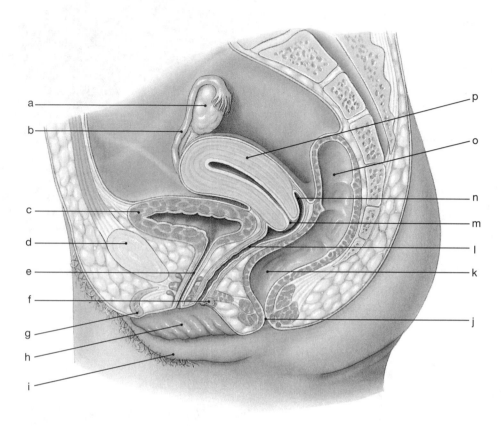

Figure 19–3 The Female Reproductive System

_____	1. Anus		_____	9. Labium majus
_____	2. Clitoris		_____	10. Ovary
_____	3. Vagina		_____	11. Labium minus
_____	4. Uterine tube		_____	12. Sigmoid colon
_____	5. Pubic symphysis		_____	13. Urethra
_____	6. Fornix		_____	14. Cervix
_____	7. Greater vestibular gland		_____	15. Urinary bladder
_____	8. Uterus		_____	16. Rectum

Identify the parts of the uterus shown in Figure 19–4. Place the corresponding letter on the line next to the appropriate label.

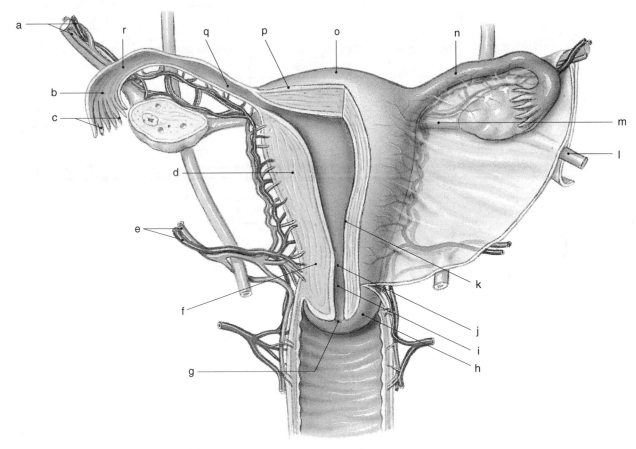

Figure 19–4 Anatomy of the Uterus

_____ 1. Fimbriae

_____ 2. Endometrium

_____ 3. Cervical canal

_____ 4. Isthmus of uterus

_____ 5. Ovarian ligament

_____ 6. Infundibulum

_____ 7. Perimetrium

_____ 8. Cervix

_____ 9. Ampulla

_____ 10. Ovarian artery and vein

_____ 11. Fundus of uterus

_____ 12. Isthmus

_____ 13. Myometrium

_____ 14. Uterine tube

_____ 15. Internal os (internal orifice)

_____ 16. Uterine artery and vein

_____ 17. Round ligament of uterus

_____ 18. Cervical os (external orifice)

SHORT ANSWER

1. Define the term *priapism* and list the medical conditions where it may be seen.

   _____

   _____

   _____

2. Discuss the pathophysiology of a ruptured ovarian cyst and list its associated symptoms.

   _____

   _____

   _____

   _____

3. Define the term *sexually transmitted disease* and list the most common types in the United States.

   _____

   _____

   _____

   _____

4. List the common complications that can occur from a woman taking combination birth control pills.

   _____

   _____

   _____

   _____

   _____

5. Discuss the clinical significance of a patient who has a testicular torsion.

   _____

   _____

   _____

   _____

20 Development and Inheritance

Chapter Objectives

Content Self-Evaluation

MULTIPLE CHOICE

_____ 1. Fertilization typically occurs in the _____.
A. lower one-third of the uterine tube   C. upper one-third of the uterine tube
B. middle one-third of the uterine tube   D. uterus

_____ 2. Fertilization involves the fusion of two haploid gametes, which produces _____.
A. a zygote with 46 chromosomes   C. a male gamete with 23 chromosomes
B. an egg with 23 chromosomes   D. a female gamete with 23 chromosomes

_____ 3. It takes sperm _____ to travel from the vagina to the point where fertilization takes place.
A. 15 to 30 minutes   C. 30 minutes to 2 hours
B. 30 to 60 minutes   D. 2 to 4 hours

_____ 4. The period of gestation in which the major organ systems begin to appear is the _____.
A. first trimester
B. second trimester
C. third trimester

_____ 5. The period of gestation in which rapid fetal growth occurs is the _____.
    A. first trimester
    B. second trimester
    C. third trimester

_____ 6. The period of gestation in which the fetus's body proportions begin to change is the _____.
    A. first trimester
    B. second trimester
    C. third trimester

_____ 7. All of the following are processes that occur during the first trimester *except* _____.
    A. cleavage and blastocyst formation   C. embryogenesis
    B. implantation   D. prostaglandin production

_____ 8. The stage where the embryo is a solid ball of cells is called the _____.
    A. blastocyst   C. trophoblast
    B. blastocoele   D. morula

_____ 9. A blastocyst is _____.
    A. a solid ball of cells   C. a hollow ball of cells
    B. part of the uterine tube   D. an enzyme released from the sperm

_____ 10. During implantation, the cells closest to the interior of the blastocyst forms a layer called the _____.
    A. syncytial trophoblast   C. cellular trophoblast
    B. lacunae   D. cytoplasm

_____ 11. During the process of gastrulation, the _____.
    A. blastocoele is formed   C. placenta is formed
    B. umbilical cord is formed   D. primary germ layers are formed

_____ 12. The primary germ layer that is in contact with the amniotic cavity is called the _____.
    A. ectoderm   C. endoderm
    B. mesoderm   D. embryonic disc

_____ 13. The primary germ layer that is a poorly organized layer of migrating cells is the _____.
    A. ectoderm   C. endoderm
    B. mesoderm   D. yolk sac

_____ 14. The primary germ layer that faces the blastocoele is called the _____.
    A. ectoderm   C. endoderm
    B. mesoderm   D. amnion

_____ 15. The extraembryonic membrane that is developed from both ectoderm and mesoderm is the _____.
    A. yolk sac   C. allantois
    B. amnion   D. chorion

_____ 16. The extraembryonic membrane that is developed from both endoderm and mesoderm is the _____.
    A. yolk sac   C. allantois
    B. amnion   D. chorion

_____ 17. The extraembryonic membrane that creates a rapid-transit system that links the embryo to the trophoblast is called the _____.
    A. yolk sac   C. allantois
    B. amnion   D. chorion

_____ 18. Which of the following hormones is a reliable indicator of pregnancy when elevated?
  A. human placental lactogen (hPL)   C. relaxin
  B. placental prolactin   D. human chorionic gonadotropin (hCG)

_____ 19. Which of the following hormones is essential for increasing the flexibility of the pubic symphysis, which permits the pelvis to expand during delivery?
  A. placental prolactin   C. human placental lactogen
  B. relaxin   D. progesterone

_____ 20. All of the following are maternal changes that occur during pregnancy *except*
  _____.
  A. maternal respiratory rates increase
  B. maternal blood volume increases
  C. mammary glands increase in size
  D. glomerular filtration rates decrease by 10 percent

_____ 21. By the end of gestation, maternal blood volume increases by _____.
  A. 10 percent   C. 50 percent
  B. 20 percent   D. 60 percent

_____ 22. Which of the following hormones decreases airway resistance during pregnancy?
  A. estrogen   C. relaxin
  B. progesterone   D. FSH

_____ 23. The correct sequence for the three stages of delivery is _____.
  A. placental, dilation, expulsion   C. expulsion, placental, dilation
  B. dilation, expulsion, placental   D. dilation, placental, expulsion

_____ 24. The dilation stage of delivery begins with _____ and ends with _____.
  A. the onset of labor, complete cervical dilation
  B. cervical dilation, delivery of the baby
  C. cervical dilation, delivery of the placenta
  D. the onset of labor, delivery of the baby

_____ 25. The dilation phase involves the dilation of the _____.
  A. uterus   C. endometrium
  B. uterine tubes   D. cervix

_____ 26. Which of the following is considered the afterbirth?
  A. fetal waste   C. amniotic fluid
  B. amniotic sac   D. placenta

_____ 27. About 70 percent of all twins are said to be fraternal. The other term for fraternal twins is _____.
  A. homozygotic   C. dizygotic
  B. monozygotic   D. heterozygotic

_____ 28. The medical term for identical twins is _____.
  A. homozygotic   C. dizygotic
  B. monozygotic   D. heterozygotic

_____ 29. The neonatal period extends from the moment of birth to _____.
  A. one year after   C. one month after
  B. six months after   D. three months after

_____ 30. The correct sequence of life stages is as follows: _____.
  A. infancy, neonatal, childhood, adolescence
  B. neonatal, infancy, maturity, adolescence
  C. neonatal, infancy, childhood, adolescence, maturity
  D. infancy, neonatal, childhood, maturity

_____ 31. All of the following are hormonal events that increase during puberty *except*
_____.
   A. an increase in gonadotropin-releasing hormone (GnRH)
   B. ovaries and testicles become more sensitive to FSH
   C. ovaries become less sensitive to LH
   D. anterior pituitary gland becomes more sensitive to the presence of GnRH

_____ 32. The characteristics from your mother or father that you express or that are seen are
called _____.
   A. genotypic traits   C. karyotypic traits
   B. phenotypic traits   D. allelic traits

_____ 33. Which of the following diseases is a connective tissue disease that is transmitted through
autosomal dominant inheritance?
   A. sickle cell disease   C. Huntington's disease
   B. Marfan's syndrome   D. cystic fibrosis

_____ 34. Which of the following diseases is characterized by abnormal bleeding due to a genetic
deficiency?
   A. sickle cell disease   C. Huntington's disease
   B. cystic fibrosis   D. hemophilia

_____ 35. Which one of the following diseases is characterized by the presence of an abnormal
form of hemoglobin?
   A. hemophilia   C. sickle cell disease
   B. cystic fibrosis   D. Huntington's disease

FILL IN THE BLANK

1. _____ is an enzyme found in the acrosomal cap of the sperm that breaks bonds
between adjacent follicle cells on the ovum.

2. _____ is the term used when fertilization by more than one sperm occurs.

3. The process when the male and female pronucleus fuse is called _____.

4. _____ is a series of cell divisions that begins immediately after fertilization.

5. _____ refers to the abnormal implantation of a fertilized egg outside of the
uterus.

6. The _____ is a temporary structure on the uterine wall that provides a site for
diffusion between the fetal and maternal circulations.

7. The first extraembryonic membrane to appear is the _____.

8. An _____ is an incision through the perineal musculature.

9. If complications arise during the delivery of a baby, the infant can be surgically removed by a
procedure called a _____.

10. If the splitting of the blastomeres is incomplete, _____ may develop.

11. Fully developed mammary glands produce a high protein secretion called
_____.

12. A naturally occurring termination of a pregnancy is often called a _____.

13. An abortion in which all of the uterine contents are expelled is called a _____.

14. Termination of a pregnancy deemed necessary by a physician is called a
_____.

15. The various forms of any one gene are called _____.

16. _____ is an autosomal recessive disease of the exocrine glands that causes production of excess mucus that may obstruct the lungs.

17. _____ is the most common viable chromosomal abnormality and ranges in frequency between 1.5 and 1.9 per 1000 births.

18. _____ is a syndrome in which the individual carries the sex chromosome pattern XXY.

19. _____ is the number one killer of pregnant females.

20. _____ occurs when blunt trauma causes the placenta to detach from the uterine wall early.

MATCHING

Match the terms in Column A with the words or phrases in Column B. Write the letter of the corresponding words or phrases in the spaces provided.

Column A

_____ 1. antepartum

_____ 2. gravidity

_____ 3. primipara

_____ 4. gestation

_____ 5. parity

_____ 6. multigravida

_____ 7. nulligravida

_____ 8. multipara

_____ 9. grand multiparity

_____ 10. postpartum

Column B

a. number of pregnancies carried to full term

b. pregnant more than once

c. never been pregnant

d. time interval prior to delivery

e. delivered more than one baby

f. given birth to first child

g. delivered more than seven babies

h. number of times a woman has been pregnant

i. time interval after delivery of the fetus

j. period of time for fetal development

Identify the stages of cleavage and blastocyst formation shown in Figure 20–1. Place the corresponding letter on the line next to the appropriate label.

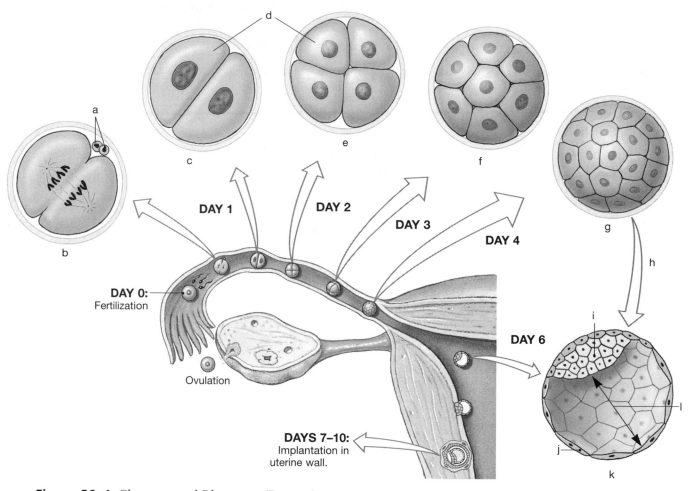

Figure 20–1 Cleavage and Blastocyst Formation

_____ 1. Advanced morula

_____ 2. Polar bodies

_____ 3. Shedding of zona pellucida

_____ 4. First cleavage division

_____ 5. Inner cell mass

_____ 6. 2-cell stage

_____ 7. Trophoblast

_____ 8. Blastomeres

_____ 9. Blastocyst

_____ 10. 4-cell stage

_____ 11. Blastocoele

_____ 12. Early morula

Identify the parts of the placenta and placental circulation shown in Figure 20–2. Place the corresponding letter on the line next to the appropriate label. _Please use each letter only once._

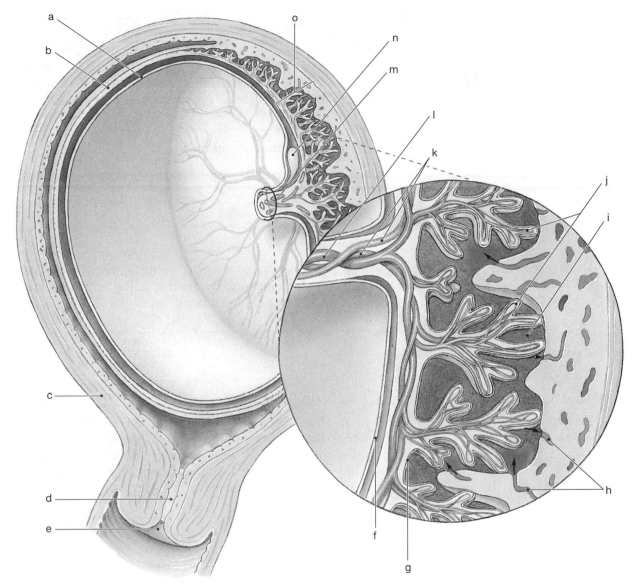

Figure 20–2 Placenta and Placental Circulation

_____ **1.** Area filled with maternal blood

_____ **2.** Amnion

_____ **3.** Cervical plug

_____ **4.** Umbilical arteries

_____ **5.** Umbilical cord (cut)

_____ **6.** Chorion

_____ **7.** Placenta

_____ **8.** Synctial trophoblast

_____ **9.** Amnion

_____ **10.** Yolk sac

_____ **11.** Umbilical vein

_____ **12.** External orifice (cervical os)

_____ **13.** Chorionic villi

_____ **14.** Maternal blood vessels

_____ **15.** Myometrium

SHORT ANSWER

1. Discuss the signs and symptoms that are seen with an ectopic pregnancy.

_____

_____

_____

_____

2. You are treating a female patient who tells you that she is 6 months pregnant. She tells you that she has two children with no miscarriages. What is the patient's gravidity and parity status?

_____

3. What type of disease is cystic fibrosis and what organs are impacted by it?

_____

_____

_____

_____

4. You are working a shift in the emergency department when a mother brings in her 10-year-old son who is complaining of excruciating pain in his leg joints. The mother tells you that he has sickle cell disease. Why would sickle cell disease cause pain in this patient's legs?

_____

_____

_____

_____

5. You stop by the scene of an automobile accident where a 24-year-old female is found lying supine on the ground. Patient tells you that she is eight months pregnant. Patient also tells you that while she was getting out of the car, she began to feel weak so she laid down on the ground. You check her blood pressure and it is low at 82/60. Other than the trauma of the automobile accident, what else could be causing this patient's blood pressure to be lower than normal?

_____

_____

_____

_____

©2008 Pearson Education, Inc.
Anatomy & Physiology for Emergency Care, 2nd ed.

Comprehensive Exam

MULTIPLE CHOICE

_____ 1. The normal human pH range of the blood ranges from _____.
   A. 7.00 to 7.35
   B. 7.35 to 7.45
   C. 7.45 to 7.55
   D. 7.00 to 7.15

_____ 2. When a red blood cell is placed in contact with a hypotonic solution, the cell will swell and potentially burst. This is referred to as _____.
   A. isotonic
   B. equaltonic
   C. crenation
   D. hemolysis

_____ 3. The layer of the epidermis that undergoes cell replication the most is the _____.
   A. subcutaneous layer
   B. dermal papillae
   C. stratum corneum
   D. stratum germinativum

_____ 4. Which of the following neurotransmitters is responsible for muscle contraction?
   A. dopamine
   B. serotonin
   C. norepinephrine
   D. acetylcholine

_____ 5. Which of the following tactile receptors are sensitive to fine touch and pressure and are found on the eyelids, lips, and fingertips?
   A. Ruffini corpuscles
   B. Meissner's corpuscles
   C. Merkel's discs
   D. lamellated corpuscles

_____ 6. _____ is the corticosteroid that is responsible for the conservation of sodium ions.
   A. Cortisol
   B. Estrogen
   C. Aldosterone
   D. Hydrocortisone

_____ 7. Which of the following equations is true regarding cardiac output?
   A. $CO = PVR \times HR$
   B. $CO = PVR \times SV$
   C. $CO = SV \times HR$
   D. $CO = EF \times HR$

_____ 8. The first line of specific defense that occurs with exposure to a pathogen is _____.
   A. B cell activation
   B. phagocytosis
   C. NK cell activation
   D. T cell activation

_____ 9. Hydrochloric acid lowers the pH of the stomach contents. Which of the following cells is responsible for secreting the hydrochloric acid?
   A. gastric pits
   B. parietal cells
   C. chief cells
   D. gastric glands

_____ 10. _____ is also called thiamine and is essential for carbohydrate metabolism.
   A. B$_1$
   B. B$_2$
   C. B$_6$
   D. B$_{12}$

_____ 11. Which of the following hormones triggers ovulation?
   A. luteinizing hormone
   B. follicle-stimulating hormone
   C. gonadotropin-releasing hormone
   D. inhibin

_____ 12. All of the following are hormonal events that increase during puberty _except_
_____.
   A. an increase in gonadotropin-releasing hormone (GnRH)
   B. ovaries and testicles become more sensitive to FSH
   C. ovaries become less sensitive to LH
   D. anterior pituitary gland becomes more sensitive to the presence of GnRH

_____ 13. The _____ plane divides the body into anterior and posterior sections.
   A. transverse
   B. midsagittal
   C. sagittal
   D. frontal

_____ 14. Which muscle tissue has intercalated discs located within the muscle?
   A. smooth
   B. skeletal
   C. voluntary
   D. cardiac

_____ 15. A rather new way to provide a route for fluid administration or medications in a life-threatening situation is the intraosseous (IO) route. The IO needle is placed into the _____ of the bone in order to provide emergency fluids or medications.
   A. periosteum
   B. diaphysis
   C. medullary cavity
   D. osteon

_____ 16. The blood-brain barrier is an essential part of isolating the brain from the general circulation. Which one of the following neuroglial cells is responsible for this?
   A. astrocytes
   B. oligodendrocytes
   C. microglia
   D. ependymal

_____ 17. The fluid found between the bony and membranous labyrinth is called _____.
   A. endolymph
   B. perilymph
   C. saccule
   D. exolymph

_____ 18. Which of the following is the best definition for polyuria?
   A. decreased urination
   B. increased urination
   C. decreased thirst
   D. increased thirst

19. When assessing a patient's blood pressure, you will normally hear Korotkoff sounds during the process. What are Korotkoff sounds?
    A. the first sound heard or the systolic pressure
    B. the sound heard when above 200 mm/Hg
    C. the sound heard as the pressure in the cuff falls below the systolic pressure
    D. the sound heard as the pressure in the cuff falls below the diastolic pressure

20. In the elderly, B cells become less active due to a reduced number of _____.
    A. suppressor T cells
    B. helper T cells
    C. NK cells
    D. antibodies

21. Because of the chemical structure of the molecule, _____ has more than 200 times the affinity of oxygen to bind with hemoglobin.
    A. carbon dioxide
    B. carbon tetrachloride
    C. carbon monoxide
    D. nitrogen

22. Which of the following segments of the nephron is impermeable to both water and solutes?
    A. proximal convoluted tubule
    B. distal convoluted tubule
    C. ascending limb of loop of Henle
    D. descending limb of loop of Henle

23. Which of the following hormones is a reliable indicator of pregnancy when elevated?
    A. human placental lactogen (hPL)
    B. placental prolactin
    C. relaxin
    D. human chorionic gonadotropin (hCG)

24. Which of the following best defines the following reaction?

$$AB \rightarrow A + B$$

    A. synthesis reaction
    B. exchange reaction
    C. decomposition reaction
    D. dehydration reaction

25. Cardiac and skeletal muscle have which of the following similarities?
    A. Both have intercalated discs.
    B. Both are single nucleated muscle cells.
    C. Both are striated.
    D. Both are under voluntary control.

26. Which of the following statements about acetylcholine (ACh) is correct?
    A. ACh breaks down molecules of cholinesterase.
    B. ACh triggers the contraction of the muscle fiber.
    C. ACh is a product of aerobic metabolism.
    D. ACh changes the permeability of the muscle to calcium.

27. Which of the following white blood cells represents around 4 percent of the total white blood cells and increase during an allergic reaction?
    A. lymphocytes
    B. neutrophils
    C. eosinophils
    D. basophils

_____ 28. The specific defense system is activated by contact with a(n) _____.
   A. antibody
   B. antigen
   C. interferon
   D. pyrogen

_____ 29. Which of the following lists the regions of the nephron in the correct order of flow?
   A. distal convoluted tubule, loop of Henle, proximal convoluted tubule, glomerular capsule
   B. proximal convoluted tubule, loop of Henle, distal convoluted tubule, glomerular capsule
   C. glomerular capsule, proximal convoluted tubule, loop of Henle, distal convoluted tubule
   D. loop of Henle, proximal convoluted tubule, distal convoluted tubule, glomerular capsule

_____ 30. The correct sequence of life stages is as follows: _____.
   A. infancy, neonatal, childhood, adolescence
   B. neonatal, infancy, maturity, adolescence
   C. neonatal, infancy, childhood, adolescence, maturity
   D. infancy, neonatal, childhood, maturity

_____ 31. When utilizing directional references, the term lateral refers to _____.
   A. toward the body's longitudinal axis
   B. away from the body's longitudinal axis
   C. toward an attached base
   D. away from an attached base

_____ 32. Which of the following best describes a third-degree burn?
   A. superficial burn with redness
   B. intense pain with limited blistering
   C. damage to all layers of the skin
   D. burn around the mouth and nose area

_____ 33. The _____ is (are) responsible for the red blood cell's ability to transport oxygen and carbon dioxide.
   A. hemoglobin
   B. leukocytes
   C. platelets
   D. hematocrit

_____ 34. Below is a list of structures that are found in the respiratory tree.
   1. bronchioles
   2. secondary bronchi
   3. alveoli
   4. alveolar ducts
   5. primary bronchi
   6. respiratory bronchioles
   7. terminal bronchioles

   Place the above structures in the correct order that air moves through the structures.
   A. 5, 2, 1, 7, 6, 4, 3
   B. 5, 2, 1, 6, 7, 4, 3
   C. 2, 5, 1, 7, 6, 4, 3
   D. 2, 5, 1, 6, 7, 3, 4

_____ 35. The pancreas is an essential organ when it comes to digestion. Not only does it release insulin and glucagon, but it also releases _____ to aid in digestion.
   A. lipases
   B. pancreatic amylase
   C. proteases
   D. All of the above.

©2008 Pearson Education, Inc.
Anatomy & Physiology for Emergency Care, 2nd ed.

_____ 36. If the intracellular fluid becomes more concentrated with respect to the extracellular fluid, water will move _____.
A. from the extracellular fluid into the cells
B. against the gradient using active transport
C. from the cell to the extracellular fluid
D. No fluid will move because the two areas are equal.

_____ 37. The most important high-energy compound in the body is _____.
A. RNA
B. DNA
C. ATP
D. H_2O

_____ 38. Which of the following involves a complete displacement of bone ends from a joint?
A. subluxation
B. fracture
C. dislocation
D. sprain

_____ 39. When the action potential of the cell jumps from node to node, it can travel much faster than if traveling through the cell. What is this process called?
A. continuous propagation
B. saltatory propagation
C. depolarization
D. repolarization

_____ 40. The area of a blood vessel that is responsible for the majority of clotting can be found in the _____.
A. tunica media
B. tunica adventitia
C. epithelial layer
D. endothelial layer

_____ 41. The most important metabolic fuel in the body is _____.
A. fructose
B. galactose
C. glucose
D. maltose

_____ 42. The right and left coronary arteries originate at the base of the _____.
A. pulmonary artery
B. superior vena cava
C. aorta
D. inferior vena cava

_____ 43. With aging comes an increase in stiffness of the chest wall and a reduction in pulmonary ventilation. This has the greatest impact on _____.
A. tidal volume
B. vital capacity
C. residual volume
D. inspiratory reserve

_____ 44. The catabolism of one fatty acid molecule generates _____ ATP molecules.
A. 72
B. 90
C. 122
D. 144

_____ 45. At which of the following ages do the primary oocytes begin meiosis?
A. three to seven months of age
B. from birth to one year of age
C. five to seven years of age
D. eleven to twelve years of age

_____ 46. Which of the following is one of the functions of the Golgi apparatus?
A. synthesizes lipids
B. controls metabolism
C. synthesizes proteins
D. packages and secretes products

_____ 47. Which of the following best describes the normal unidirectional flow of an impulse through a neuron?
A. axon, cell body, dendrite
B. dendrite, axon, cell body
C. dendrite, cell body, axon
D. cell body, dendrite, axon

_____ 48. Which of the following is responsible for recharging the energy-spent ADP back to the high-energy ATP?
A. cAMP
B. creatine phosphate
C. glucose
D. oxygen

_____ 49. A reflex that has a direct connection from the sensory neuron to the motor neuron is referred to as a _____ reflex.
A. disynaptic
B. monosynaptic
C. stretch
D. flexor

_____ 50. Which two hormones are released directly into the circulation at the posterior pituitary gland?
A. epinephrine and norepinephrine
B. thyroid and parathyroid
C. ADH and oxytocin
D. growth hormone and thyroid hormone

_____ 51. The subclavian artery immediately branches into the _____.
A. brachial artery
B. radial artery
C. ulnar artery
D. axillary artery

_____ 52. The breakdown of carbohydrates generates approximately_____ calories per gram of energy.
A. 2
B. 4
C. 9
D. 12

_____ 53. The dilation stage of delivery begins with _____ and ends with _____.
A. the onset of labor, complete cervical dilation
B. cervical dilation, delivery of the baby
C. cervical dilation, delivery of the placenta
D. the onset of labor, delivery of the baby

_____ 54. _____ describes when a stimulus produces a response that reinforces the original stimulus.
   A. Control center
   B. Negative feedback
   C. Positive feedback
   D. Homeostasis

_____ 55. The outer most layer of the skin is called the _____.
   A. dermis papillae
   B. subcutaneous layer
   C. stratum corneum
   D. stratum germinativum

_____ 56. Which of the following is a type of fracture in which the fracture site has multiple bone fragments?
   A. torus
   B. transverse
   C. oblique
   D. comminuted

_____ 57. The hair cells of the cochlear duct are located in the _____.
   A. organ of Corti
   B. tectorial membrane
   C. tympanic duct
   D. basilar membrane

_____ 58. Which of the following hormones stimulates thirst?
   A. renin
   B. aldosterone
   C. angiotensin I
   D. angiotensinogen

_____ 59. Which of the following antibodies is found in exocrine secretions like tears and saliva?
   A. IgA
   B. IgE
   C. IgD
   D. IgM

_____ 60. The movement of air in and out of the lungs is dependent upon _____.
   A. pressure differences between the lungs and the atmosphere
   B. pressure differences between the diaphragm and the pleural space
   C. pressure differences between the capillaries and alveoli
   D. pressure differences between the atmosphere and the inspiratory reserve volume

_____ 61. Phenylketonuria is an inherited disease that prevents the conversion of the amino acid phenylalanine to the amino acid _____.
   A. valine
   B. leucine
   C. lysine
   D. tyrosine

_____ 62. During menopause, there is a decline in the circulating concentrations of _____.
   A. GnRH
   B. FSH
   C. LH
   D. estrogen

_____ 63. Where are osteocytes located within the structure of the bone?
A. periosteum
B. canaliculi
C. lacunae
D. lamella

_____ 64. Which of the following ions are responsible for binding to the troponin, which allows for muscle contraction?
A. sodium
B. potassium
C. magnesium
D. calcium

_____ 65. Erythropoietin is a hormone that is released from the _____ when oxygen concentrations decrease.
A. brain
B. liver
C. kidneys
D. bone marrow

_____ 66. During the plateau phase, _____ release causes the cardiac muscle to contract.
A. calcium
B. sodium
C. potassium
D. chloride

_____ 67. Which of the following is the correct order of swallowing phases?
A. oral, esophageal, pharyngeal
B. oral, pharyngeal, esophageal
C. pharyngeal, oral, esophageal
D. pharyngeal, esophageal, oral

_____ 68. An angiotensin-converting enzyme is responsible for converting _____.
A. angiotensinogen to angiotensin I
B. angiotensinogen to angiotensin II
C. angiotensin I to angiotensin II
D. angiotensin II to angiotensin I

_____ 69. Which of the following phases occurs when the endometrium prepares for the arrival of the developing embryo?
A. secretory phase
B. proliferative phase
C. follicular phase
D. ovarian phase

_____ 70. The thoracic body cavity is subdivided into the _____.
A. cranial and spinal cavities
B. abdominal and pelvic cavities
C. thoracic and abdominal cavities
D. pleural and pericardial cavities

_____ 71. An injury to the skin where a flap of tissue is torn loose or completely off is referred to as a(n) _____.
A. amputation
B. abrasion
C. avulsion
D. laceration

©2008 Pearson Education, Inc.
Anatomy & Physiology for Emergency Care, 2nd ed.

_____ 72. Organophosphate insecticides like sarin gas have been used in previous terrorist attacks. Which of the following is the principle action of organophosphate poisons?
   A. decreases acetylcholine release
   B. deactivates acetylcholinesterase
   C. increases acetylcholinesterase release
   D. deactivates acetylcholine

_____ 73. Hormones bind to cell membrane receptors and do not have a direct effect on the cell. Therefore, hormones are considered _____.
   A. first messengers
   B. second messengers
   C. third messengers
   D. fourth messengers

_____ 74. The movement of carbon dioxide and oxygen in and out of the alveoli occurs by _____.
   A. osmosis
   B. active transport
   C. facilitated transport
   D. diffusion

_____ 75. During the complete catabolism of one glucose molecule, a cell will gain _____ ATP molecules.
   A. 30
   B. 32
   C. 34
   D. 36

_____ 76. During implantation, the cells closest to the interior of the blastocyst forms a layer called the _____.
   A. syncytial trophoblast
   B. lacunae
   C. cellular trophoblast
   D. cytoplasm

_____ 77. Ions with a positive charge are called _____.
   A. electrons
   B. cations
   C. anions
   D. protons

_____ 78. Cardiac and smooth muscle have which of the following similarities?
   A. Both are under voluntary control.
   B. Both are under involuntary control.
   C. Both have intercalated discs.
   D. Both are multinucleated cells.

_____ 79. Which of the following ions rushes into the muscle cell to spread the action potential?
   A. calcium
   B. sodium
   C. potassium
   D. chloride

_____ 80. The outermost layer of the eye, which consists of the sclera and cornea, is called the
_____.
A. anterior cavity
B. fibrous tunic
C. vascular tunic
D. neural tunic

_____ 81. The correct order through the cardiac conducting system is _____.
A. SA node, AV node, Purkinje fibers, right and left bundle branches
B. AV node, SA node, bundle of His, Purkinje fibers, right and left bundle branches
C. SA node, AV node, bundle of His, right and left bundle branches, Purkinje fibers
D. AV node, SA node, bundle of His, right and left bundle branches, Purkinje fibers

_____ 82. The activation of plasminogen produces an enzyme, which digests the fibrin strands of the clot. This enzyme is called _____.
A. prothrombin
B. thrombin
C. plasmin
D. fibrinogen

_____ 83. Which of the following is the normal path that food takes through the digestive tract?
A. oral cavity, esophagus, stomach, pharynx, large intestine, small intestine, anus, rectum
B. oral cavity, pharynx, esophagus, stomach, small intestine, large intestine, rectum, anus
C. pharynx, oral cavity, esophagus, stomach, small intestine, large intestine, rectum, anus
D. pharynx, oral cavity, esophagus, stomach, large intestine, small intestine, rectum, anus

_____ 84. The juxtaglomerular apparatus is the endocrine structure that secretes _____.
A. renin and angiotensin I
B. angiotensin I and erythropoietin
C. ADH and renin
D. renin and erythropoietin

_____ 85. When utilizing directional references, the term proximal refers to _____.
A. toward the body's longitudinal axis
B. away from the body's longitudinal axis
C. toward an attached base
D. away from an attached base

_____ 86. The movement of water across a cell membrane occurs by _____.
A. primary active transport
B. secondary active transport
C. facilitated diffusion
D. osmosis

_____ 87. Which of the following is considered the primary complication of scurvy?
A. increase in osteoclast production
B. decrease in osteoclast production
C. increase in osteoblast production
D. decrease in osteoblast production

©2008 Pearson Education, Inc.
Anatomy & Physiology for Emergency Care, 2nd ed.

_____ 88. Patients with diabetes may suffer from polydipsia. Which of the following is the best definition for polydipsia?
  A. decreased urination
  B. increased urination
  C. decreased thirst
  D. increased thirst

_____ 89. The valve that is located between the left atrium and left ventricle is called the _____ valve.
  A. aortic
  B. pulmonic
  C. mitral
  D. tricuspid

_____ 90. Which of the following is the hormone that stimulates the gallbladder to release bile?
  A. gastrin
  B. secretin
  C. cholecystokinin (CCK)
  D. gastric inhibitory peptide (GIP)

_____ 91. Which of the following is a function of the mitochondria?
  A. synthesizes proteins
  B. synthesizes lipids
  C. produces ATP
  D. controls metabolism

_____ 92. Osteocytes can be found within small pockets of the bone called the _____.
  A. lamellae
  B. canaliculi
  C. lacunae
  D. central canal

_____ 93. Which of the following is the correct route sperm would take to exit the body?
  A. epididymis, ejaculatory duct, ductus deferens, urethra
  B. epididymis, ductus deferens, ejaculatory duct, urethra
  C. ductus deferens, epididymis, urethra, ejaculatory duct
  D. ejaculatory duct, epididymis, urethra, ductus deferens

_____ 94. The three classes of lymphocytes are _____.
  A. monocytes, basophils, eosinophils
  B. T cells, B cells, NK cells
  C. red blood cells, platelets, white blood cells
  D. neutrophils, eosinophils, basophils

_____ 95. The difference between the systolic pressure and the diastolic pressure is called the _____.
  A. pulsus alternans
  B. pulsus paradoxsus
  C. pulse pressure
  D. blood pressure

_____ 96. Which of the following receptors when stimulated will cause analgesia?
  A. mu-2
  B. beta
  C. sigma
  D. epsilon

_____ 97. Shingles is a viral syndrome that is also referred to as _____.
   A. herpes varicella
   B. herpes zoster
   C. herpes simplex
   D. herpes complex

_____ 98. When a cell is selective and only allows certain substances to cross it, the membrane is said to be _____.
   A. impermeable
   B. permeable
   C. selectively permeable
   D. passively permeable

_____ 99. If the normal resting membrane potential is −70 mV, what would the membrane potential be if the membrane was hyperpolarized?
   A. +5 mV
   B. −65 mV
   C. −80 mV
   D. +70 mV

_____ 100. In fetal circulation, there is an opening between the pulmonary artery and the aorta to allow for oxygenated blood to come from the mother to the baby. The hole is called the _____.
   A. fossa ovalis
   B. foramen magnum
   C. ductus arteriosus
   D. ligamentum arteriosum

ANSWER KEY

Chapter 1

MULTIPLE CHOICE

1. B	3. C	5. D	7. B	9. C
2. C	4. C	6. D	8. C	10. B

FILL IN THE BLANK

1. Metabolism
2. Pathology or pathological physiology
3. cell physiology
4. anatomy, physiology
5. cell
6. nervous
7. lymphatic
8. alveoli
9. homeostasis
10. thoracic, abdominopelvic

TRUE/FALSE

1. False	4. True	7. True	10. False
2. False	5. True	8. True	
3. True	6. False	9. True	

LABELING EXERCISE 1–1

1. A	7. B	13. M	19. AA	25. X
2. C	8. U	14. V	20. G	26. CC
3. D	9. L	15. H	21. T	27. O
4. K	10. E	16. P	22. Z	28. DD
5. N	11. R	17. Y	23. J	29. S
6. Q	12. F	18. I	24. BB	30. W

LABELING EXERCISE 1–2

1. B	4. D	7. C	10. G	13. A
2. F	5. M	8. H	11. E	
3. I	6. J	9. L	12. K	

LABELING EXERCISE 1–3

1. C or E	4. B	7. I	10. D or F
2. D or F	5. K	8. C or E	11. G
3. H	6. A	9. L	12. J

LABELING EXERCISE 1–4

1. B	3. G	5. I	7. F	9. H
2. D	4. C	6. E	8. A	

LABELING EXERCISE 1–5

1. D	3. F	5. A	7. G
2. B	4. H	6. E	8. C

SHORT ANSWER

1. Anatomy is the study of the internal and external structures and the physical relationship between body organs or systems. Anatomy can be studied broadly at the gross anatomy level, or locally can be divided into regional or systemic anatomy. Each level looks at the physical structure of the organ and its relationship to other organs within the same system or different systems.

   Physiology is the study of how living organisms perform their vital functions. Human physiology is the study of the function of the human body. Physiology can be broken down into more specific areas of physiologic functions to include cell physiology or even cardiovascular physiology.

2. Correct answers may include the following: Homeostasis refers to a stable internal environment inside the body. The body will modify physiologic systems to help maintain homeostasis. If the temperature begins to fall, the blood flow to the skin and extremities decreases. The sweat gland activity also decreases. If this response does not cause the internal temperature to rise, the skeletal muscle will begin to shiver to help increase the core body temperature. Once the internal core temperature begins to rise, the muscle stops generating heat through shivering, the blood flow to the skin and extremities increases, and sweat gland activity returns to normal.

3. The 10-year-old female patient has swelling on the lateral side of her right ankle with swelling also found on the medial side of the right lower leg proximal to the ankle.

Chapter 2

MULTIPLE CHOICE

1. C	4. C	7. B	10. B	13. C
2. C	5. C	8. B	11. B	14. C
3. B	6. C	9. C	12. C	15. A

FILL IN THE BLANK

1. ionic
2. Catabolism
3. Anabolism
4. decrease
5. Enzymes
6. inorganic
7. pH
8. Glycogen
9. polysaccharides
10. unsaturated
11. peptide
12. adenine, guanine, thymine, cytosine
13. uracil
14. energy
15. adenosine monophosphate or AMP

MATCHING

1. H	3. F	5. A	7. J	9. B
2. D	4. G	6. C	8. E	10. I

LABELING EXERCISE 2–1

1. B	2. A	3. C

LABELING EXERCISE 2–2

1. D, F, or I	4. A, G, or H	7. C or E
2. D, F, or I	5. A, G, or H	8. A, G, or H
3. B	6. C or E	9. D, F, or I

SHORT ANSWER

1. Hydrolysis reactions utilize a large molecule and water. Hydrolysis is a chemical process in which a molecule is broken into two parts by the addition of a molecule of water. In the process of the reaction, the components of the water (H + OH) are added to the broken ends or fragments of the reaction.

Condensation or dehydration reactions are the formation of a complex molecule by the removal of water.

2. The four classes of organic compounds are carbohydrates, lipids, proteins, and nucleic acids.

Carbohydrates are organic molecules comprised of carbon, hydrogen, and oxygen. Sugars and starches are examples of carbohydrates.

Lipids are also comprised of carbon, hydrogen, and oxygen. The big difference between lipids and carbohydrates is that lipids are made up of less oxygen and may include phosphorus, nitrogen, or sulfur. Lipids store more than twice the amount of energy or calories than carbohydrates. Examples of lipids are fatty acids, steroids, and phospholipids.

Proteins are the most abundant of all organic compounds. There are roughly 400,000 different kinds of proteins in the body, but examples include hemoglobin, keratin, myoglobin, and enzymes.

Nucleic acids store and process genetic information at the molecular level. The two classes of nucleic acids are deoxyribonucleic acid (DNA) and ribonucleic acid (RNA). DNA determines our inherited characteristics. RNA comes in more than one form and is responsible for manufacturing proteins.

3. Both DNA and RNA are composed of repeating units of nucleotides. Each nucleotide consists of a sugar, a phosphate, and a nitrogenous base. The sugar in DNA is deoxyribose. The sugar in RNA is ribose, the same as deoxyribose but with one more OH (oxygen-hydrogen atom combination called a hydroxyl group). Another difference between the two is DNA is the only nucleic acid that utilizes thymine as a nitrogenous base, while RNA utilizes uracil. RNA also differs because of the much greater variety of nucleic acid bases available to make the numerous proteins that are needed.

4. ATP is comprised of three components, the first of which is nucleotide adenosine monophosphate, which is a combination of sugar, adenine, and a phosphate. The other components are two phosphate groups. The greatest amount of energy is held in the bond between the second and third phosphate group.

5. Normally, ATP is continuously generated in cells. When little to no ATP is available, numerous cell functions, including muscle contraction and synthesis of proteins, cannot occur.

Chapter 3

MULTIPLE CHOICE

1. C	4. D	7. D	10. A	13. D
2. D	5. A	8. C	11. C	14. C
3. B	6. B	9. A	12. C	15. C

FILL IN THE BLANK

1. cell
2. cell membrane
3. Lysosomes
4. Golgi apparatus
5. hypotonic
6. active transport
7. sperm
8. ribosomes
9. gene
10. 23

11. nucleus
12. transcription
13. meiosis
14. metaphase
15. malignant

MATCHING

1. H	3. C	5. I	7. G	9. F
2. B	4. A	6. D	8. J	10. E

LABELING EXERCISE 3–1

1. G	4. J	7. K	10. F
2. A	5. H	8. E *or* I	11. E *or* I
3. D	6. B	9. C	

LABELING EXERCISE 3–2

1. H	5. D	9. A	13. E	17. C
2. P	6. M	10. R	14. B	18. N
3. F	7. O	11. I	15. J	19. G
4. K	8. Q	12. S	16. L	

LABELING EXERCISE 3–3

1. D	3. G	5. C	7. F
2. B	4. E	6. A	

SHORT ANSWER

1. The first function of the cell membrane is physical isolation. The membrane provides a barrier between the inside and outside of the cell. Without this barrier, muscles could not contract and neurons would not be able to conduct information from the brain to the body. This barrier or separation is essential to maintain homeostasis.

The second function is the regulation of exchange with the environment. The cell membrane helps control what goes inside and outside the cell.

The third function is sensitivity. The cell membrane has receptors that enable the cell to recognize and respond to specific molecules in its environment.

The last function of the cell membrane is structural support. Specialized connections between cell membranes, or between membranes and extracellular materials, give tissues a stable structure.

2. Osmosis is the movement of water from an area of low solute concentration to an area of high solute concentration. Water can easily pass from one side of a membrane to the other. In cases where solute or particles are too big to move through diffusion, water can move to change the concentration on both sides of the membrane.

Diffusion is the movement of solute or particles from an area of high concentration to an area of low concentration. This requires no energy spent by the cells for this to occur. An example of diffusion would be how oxygen and carbon dioxide are exchanged between the alveoli and the capillaries in the lungs.

3. A solution that contains 4.5 percent normal saline is considered hypertonic. The normal or isotonic concentration of normal saline is 0.9 percent. Since 4.5 percent has a greater tonicity or osmotic pressure, fluid is pulled from the cell, which causes the cell to shrink in size. The other term for this is crenation.

4. UAA is one of the three stop codons recognized during translation to stop the synthesis of the

protein. The other two stop codons are UGA and UAG. When either one of the three stop codons are presented by the transfer RNA (tRNA), the process of translation for that protein is stopped and the protein is transferred to the Golgi apparatus for further packaging.

5. DNA technology has already played an important role in medicine. The development of synthetic insulin for diabetic patients or the development of clot-busting anti-stroke drugs like Activase has already made a huge impact in patient care. Further technology may even lead us to information needed to develop new and better drugs with fewer adverse side effects which will make the drugs safer and easier to use.

Chapter 4

MULTIPLE CHOICE

1. B	4. B	7. C	10. C	13. B
2. B	5. B	8. B	11. D	14. C
3. C	6. D	9. A	12. C	15. D

FILL IN THE BLANK

1. Endocrine
2. tight junction
3. simple epithelium
4. Simple cuboidal
5. Pseudostratified columnar epithelial
6. stratified squamous epithelial
7. Mast cells
8. Collagen
9. Marfan's
10. Mucous
11. Loose connective
12. Hyaline
13. Menisci
14. Synaptic terminals
15. osteoporosis

MATCHING

1. C	3. B	5. F	7. A	9. H
2. D	4. G	6. E	8. J	10. I

LABELING EXERCISE 4–1

1. C	5. B	9. L	13. K
2. E	6. J	10. A	14. F
3. I	7. G	11. M	15. P
4. N	8. O	12. H	16. D

LABELING EXERCISE 4–2

1. B	2. D	3. E	4. C	5. A

SHORT ANSWER

1. Macrophages are found within the matrix of the connective tissue. Macrophages phagocytize damaged cells or pathogens that enter the tissue. Macrophages can release chemicals that attract additional macrophages to the area. This helps mobilize the immune system to defend against a pathogen or foreign substance.

2. During rapid deceleration blunt trauma, such as a motor vehicle accident, the descending portion of the aorta continues to move forward after the vehicle stops. This can cause the ligamentum arteriosum to tear through a section of the aorta, which causes massive blood loss and, in most cases, death.

3. Bone is comprised of mostly calcium compounds and flexible collagen fibers. The bone cells or osteocytes are found within the lacunae of the bone and receive blood for repair and growth.

Cartilage is comprised of chondrocytes also found within the lacunae of the matrix within the cartilage. Cartilage is more gelatinous than bone and is avascular. There are no blood vessels within the capsule or structure of the cartilage. This lack of blood supply limits repair capabilities of the cartilage.

Chapter 5

MULTIPLE CHOICE

1. D	4. C	7. C	10. C	13. C
2. C	5. B	8. D	11. B	14. B
3. D	6. C	9. C	12. C	15. B

FILL IN THE BLANK

1. Albinism
2. carotene, melanin
3. vitamin D_3
4. basal cell carcinoma
5. fissure
6. Petechiae or Purpura
7. Sebum
8. apocrine glands
9. Atopic eczema
10. abrasion
11. crush injury
12. first-degree
13. Bilirubin
14. transdermal
15. Melanocytes

MATCHING

1. C	3. A	5. B	7. J	9. G
2. E	4. F	6. D	8. I	10. H

LABELING EXERCISE 5–1

1. D	5. P	9. O	13. K	17. E
2. L	6. M	10. H	14. C	
3. B	7. A	11. Q	15. I	
4. G	8. J	12. F	16. N	

LABELING EXERCISE 5–2

1. C	3. E	5. A	7. B	9. D
2. F	4. G	6. I	8. H	

LABELING EXERCISE 5–3

1. C	4. L	7. K	10. M	13. F
2. H	5. B	8. G	11. D	
3. E	6. J	9. A	12. I	

SHORT ANSWER

1. A predetermined amount of a medication is placed into a transdermal adhesive patch. These drugs must be lipid-soluble in order to penetrate the skin. Alternatively, the drug can be mixed with a solvent that is highly lipid-soluble. The resultant mixture is absorbed through the skin. The patch is applied to the skin, and the drug is slowly absorbed. Once the drug has penetrated the cell membranes in the *stratum corneum* and enters the underlying tissues, it is absorbed into the circulation.

2. A second-degree burn is also called a partial thickness burn. The epidermis is burned through and the dermis is damaged. There is usually intense pain and blistering. The blisters develop as plasma and interstitial fluids are released into the skin and elevate the top layer. An example of a second-degree burn is a scalding burn from boiling water.

3. Skin cancers are the most common form of cancer, and they include basal cell carcinoma, squamous cell carcinoma, and melanoma.

The most common skin cancer is basal cell carcinoma, which originates in the stratum germinativum (basal) layer. Less common is squamous cell carcinoma, which involves more superficial layers of epidermal cells. Metastasis seldom occurs in either cancer, and most people survive these cancers. The usual treatment involves surgical removal of the tumor. The most common cause of skin cancer is exposure to UV radiation from the sun.

Melanomas are extremely dangerous. A melanoma usually begins from a mole but may appear anywhere in the body. Cancerous melanocytes grow rapidly and metastasize through the lymphatic system. The outlook for long-term survival depends on when the condition is detected and treated. Avoiding exposure to UV radiation in sunlight (especially during the middle of the day) and using a sunblock (not a tanning oil) would largely prevent all three forms of cancer.

4. When stimulated, the arrector pili muscle pulls on the follicle, forcing the hair to stand up. Contraction may be caused by emotional states (such as fear or rage) or a response to cold, which produces "goose bumps."

5. Correct answers may include any three of the following: protection, temperature maintenance, synthesis and storage of nutrients, sensory reception, and excretion/secretion through integumentary glands.

Chapter 6

MULTIPLE CHOICE

1. C	7. C	13. C	19. D	25. B
2. A	8. C	14. C	20. B	26. C
3. B	9. B	15. C	21. C	27. B
4. D	10. C	16. C	22. C	28. D
5. C	11. D	17. B	23. D	29. B
6. C	12. D	18. C	24. B	30. C

FILL IN THE BLANK

1. Tendons
2. osteocytes
3. Osteoblasts
4. osteon
5. Osteoclasts
6. epiphyseal
7. A, C
8. spiral
9. Scurvy
10. axial
11. sphenoid
12. maxillary bones
13. 12
14. 12
15. fontanels
16. odontoid process
17. xiphoid process
18. olecranon
19. wrist
20. ilium, ischium, pubis
21. femur
22. calcaneus
23. hinge
24. freely movable
25. menisci

MATCHING

Group A

1. G	3. J	5. C	7. F	9. B
2. E	4. D	6. H	8. I	10. A

Group B

1. I	3. H	5. F	7. D	9. J
2. C	4. G	6. B	8. A	10. E

LABELING EXERCISE 6–1

1. C	4. J	7. I	10. B
2. K	5. G	8. D	11. H
3. E	6. A	9. F	

LABELING EXERCISE 6–2

1. F	3. H	5. J	7. I	9. C
2. B	4. D	6. A	8. E	10. G

LABELING EXERCISE 6–3

1. L or O	8. U	15. Y	22. I
2. Q	9. H	16. K	23. T
3. C	10. D	17. E	24. N
4. J	11. W	18. X	25. F
5. G	12. A	19. P	
6. S	13. R	20. B	
7. O or L	14. M	21. V	

LABELING EXERCISE 6–4

1. L	6. P	11. F	16. I	21. K
2. N	7. C	12. U	17. O	
3. J	8. T	13. A	18. D	
4. H	9. G	14. S	19. M	
5. E	10. R	15. Q	20. B	

LABELING EXERCISE 6–5

1. L	6. H	11. U	16. V	20. G
2. N	7. S	12. I	17. A	21. C
3. D	8. B	13. T	18. R	22. K
4. J	9. F	14. O	19. M	
5. P	10. Q	15. E		

LABELING EXERCISE 6–6

1. B	2. E	3. C	4. A	5. D

LABELING EXERCISE 6–7

1. E	3. D	5. C
2. B	4. A	6. F

LABELING EXERCISE 6–8

1. E	3. F	5. G	7. H
2. A	4. B	6. C	8. D

LABELING EXERCISE 6–9

1. G	4. E	7. C	10. A	13. J
2. B	5. K	8. O	11. N	14. H
3. I	6. M	9. L	12. F	15. D

LABELING EXERCISE 6–10

1. E	3. F	5. G	7. H	9. I
2. A	4. B	6. C	8. D	

LABELING EXERCISE 6–11

1. E	3. F	5. G	7. H
2. A	4. B	6. C	8. D

LABELING EXERCISE 6–12

1. J	5. B	9. K	13. D
2. H	6. N	10. A	14. I
3. E	7. G or M	11. G or M	15. C
4. L	8. O	12. F	

LABELING EXERCISE 6–13

1. F	4. B	7. I	10. E
2. A	5. H	8. D	11. K
3. G	6. C	9. J	

SHORT ANSWER

1. A tendon is a band of tough, inelastic fibers that connect muscle to bone. Ligaments are a sheet or band of tough, fibrous tissue that connect bones or cartilages to another bone at a joint.

2. The five functions of the skeletal system are structural support; storage of calcium and lipids; blood cell production; protection of vital organs; and leverage in connection with muscle.

3. The four types of bones are the long bones (e.g., femur, humerus); short bones (e.g., carpal and tarsal bones); flat bones (e.g., parietal bones of the skull, scapulae, ribs); and irregular bones (e.g., vertebrae of the spinal column).

4. The epiphyseal plate is the growth plate of the bone. This plate is made of cartilage. The length of the shaft of the bone continues to grow with new cartilage as the older cartilage is replaced with bone. Damage to this process could affect the future growth of the bone. Fractures through the growth plate (Harris-Salter fractures) require surgical intervention.

5. The four steps of bone injury and repair are the following:

Step 1: Begins with the fracture or damage to the bone. Blood vessels are broken and bleeding occurs in the area of the injury. Thus, lack of blood supply leads to some osteocyte death.

Step 2: Cells within the periosteum and endosteum begin to undergo mitosis. These daughter cells migrate to the area of injury and internal and external thickening (callus) of the bone occurs.

Step 3: Osteoblasts replace the central cartilage portion of the callus with spongy bone. The ends of the fracture can now withstand normal stresses from muscle contractions.

Step 4: Remodeling of the spongy bone at the fracture site continues for a period of four months to well over a year. When remodeling of the bone is complete, the callus will be gone and living compact bone will remain. The only way to tell a fracture was ever there is the bone may be slightly thicker at the fracture site.

Chapter 7

MULTIPLE CHOICE

1. C	8. B	15. C	22. D	29. D
2. A	9. D	16. C	23. C	30. C
3. B	10. D	17. B	24. A	31. A
4. A	11. D	18. D	25. D	32. B
5. C	12. A	19. C	26. B	33. B
6. B	13. C	20. B	27. D	34. B
7. A	14. B	21. D	28. C	35. C

ORDERING EXERCISE

1. C	3. D	5. H	7. I	9. G
2. E	4. A	6. F	8. B	

FILL IN THE BLANK

1. Tendons
2. sarcoplasm
3. sarcoplasmic reticulum
4. Actin, myosin
5. synaptic cleft
6. Rhabdomyolysis
7. tropomyosin
8. Tropomyosin
9. relaxation
10. botulism
11. Creatine phosphokinase

12. Succinylcholine (Anectine)
13. origin
14. frontalis
15. masseter
16. diaphragm
17. biceps femoris, semitendinosus, semimembranosus
18. smaller in diameter
19. carpal tunnel
20. Polio

MATCHING

Group A

1. H	3. C	5. I	7. J	9. D
2. E	4. G	6. A	8. B	10. F

Group B

1. C	3. E	5. J	7. I	9. G
2. D	4. H	6. A	8. B	10. F

LABELING EXERCISE 7–1

1. A	3. B	5. C	7. D	9. E
2. F	4. G	6. H	8. I	

LABELING EXERCISE 7–2

1. E	3. A	5. D
2. F	4. B	6. C

LABELING EXERCISE 7–3

1. BB	9. II	17. E	25. V	33. J
2. S	10. D	18. FF	26. O	34. Z
3. DD	11. MM	19. I	27. GG	35. R
4. F	12. U	20. AA	28. L	36. N
5. Q	13. B	21. P	29. EE	37. X
6. A	14. KK	22. LL	30. G	38. T
7. Y	15. M	23. H	31. CC	39. C
8. K	16. HH	24. JJ	32. W	

LABELING EXERCISE 7–4

1. K	7. Y	13. CC	19. L	25. S
2. W	8. N	14. M	20. D	26. I
3. E	9. V	15. A	21. X	27. C
4. R	10. F	16. T	22. Q	28. U
5. P	11. BB	17. J	23. G	29. O
6. B	12. H	18. AA	24. Z	

SHORT ANSWER

1. The three types of muscle tissue are skeletal, smooth and cardiac.

   Skeletal muscle is a multi-nucleated, voluntary muscle that is striated. Examples of functions include:
   a. movement of the skeleton
   b. maintain posture and position
   c. support soft tissues
   d. maintain body temperature
   e. entrances and exits (encircle openings to digestive and urinary tracts)

   Smooth muscle is a single-nucleated, involuntary muscle cell that is nonstriated. It is found within almost every organ in the body. Examples of the functions include:
   a. maintain organ size and dimension
   b. regulate lumen diameter
   c. elasticity
   d. rhythmic peristaltic movement

   Cardiac muscle has some attributes of smooth muscle and some of skeletal muscle. Cardiac muscle is single-nucleated, striated muscle but is involuntary. Cardiac muscle is the only muscle with intercalated discs. These discs allow for an impulse to travel from muscle cell to muscle cell in a quick, organized fashion. Examples of the functions include:

   a. contraction of the atria and ventricles of the heart

   b. maintain rhythmic activity of the heart

   c. contract to provide the cardiac output needed to perfuse the body

2. Approximately six hours after death (the time varies depending on environmental temperature), the skeletal muscles have depleted all remaining glucose and ATP molecules. Waste products, primarily metabolic acids, accumulate. After the ATP is gone, the sarcoplasmic reticulum cannot remove calcium ions from the sarcoplasm. Then, myosin fibers cannot separate from actin fibers, and rigor mortis, which is a sustained contraction, sets in. The smaller muscles, usually those of the jaw, are affected first. Eventually, the entire body is affected. Finally, 12–24 hours later, lysosomal enzymes from the muscle cells break down the contracted myofilaments, and the muscles relax.

3. The nine steps to skeletal muscle contraction are as follows:

   a. The arrival of the action potential at the synaptic terminal. This is the impulse that made its way from the thalamus down the craniosacral or efferent pathway.

   b. The acetylcholine that is released from the vesicles releases from the motor-end plate of the neuron into the synaptic cleft.

   c. The acetylcholine binds to receptors found on the sarcolemma. This changes the permeability of the membrane to sodium ions. As the sodium enters the sarcolemma, this produces the action potential in the sarcolemma.

   d. The action potential spreads over the entire surface of the sarcolemma, which causes the sarcoplasmic reticulum to release its own stores of calcium ions.

   e. The calcium ions bind to the troponin complex sites found on the actin filaments. This removes the tropomyosin, which keeps the actin and myosin separated.

   f. The myosin cross-bridge forms and attaches to the exposed active sites on the actin or thin filament.

   g. The attached myosin head pivots toward the center of the sarcomere and the ADP and phosphate group are released from the site. This is sometimes called a ratcheting of the head, which causes the actin and myosin filaments to slide over each other or contract. This step requires energy that was stored in the myosin molecule. This process is called the sliding filament theory.

   h. The cross-bridges detach when the myosin head binds another ATP molecule. This is considered relaxation of the muscle.

   i. The detached myosin head is reactivated as it splits the ATP and captures the energy held in the phosphate bond.

4. Myasthenia gravis is an autoimmune disease characterized by muscle weakness and fatigue. Antibodies against acetylcholine receptors impair the function of the receptor and prevent acetylcholine from binding to it. The signs and symptoms typically begin with weakness in the eye muscles and drooping eyelids. Facial muscles also become weakened. Difficulties swallowing or even holding up the head are possible signs of the disease. Treatment is based on using drugs that will inhibit the enzyme that breaks down acetylcholine at the neuromuscular junction. Tensilon or neostigmine are drugs that inhibit cholinesterase, which will increase the amount of acetylcholine at the neuromuscular junction and allow for muscle contraction.

5. Tetanus is caused by a bacteria *Clostridium tetani*. This bacteria can be found around rusty nails and old metal. *Clostridium tetani* can only live in tissues that contain very low oxygen levels. Deep puncture-style injuries pose the greatest risk of exposure. The bacteria releases a powerful toxin that suppresses the mechanism that regulates motor neuron activity. This causes sustained, powerful contraction of skeletal muscles throughout the body. Most common early complaints of tetanus are headache, muscle stiffness, and difficulty swallowing. It becomes more and more difficult to open the mouth, hence the name "lockjaw." The best treatment is usually the human tetanus immune globulin antibody.

Chapter 8

MULTIPLE CHOICE

1. D	10. B	19. B	28. B	37. B
2. C	11. A	20. B	29. C	38. C
3. D	12. B	21. A	30. C	39. B
4. C	13. C	22. B	31. B	40. C
5. C	14. B	23. B	32. B	41. B
6. A	15. C	24. B	33. B	42. B
7. C	16. C	25. D	34. C	43. D
8. B	17. D	26. C	35. C	44. D
9. D	18. A	27. B	36. C	45. C

FILL IN THE BLANK

1. neuron
2. afferent
3. Neuroglial
4. multipolar
5. position, movement
6. Oligodendrocytes
7. Sodium
8. all-or-none
9. neuromuscular junction
10. nodes of Ranvier
11. cholinergic synapses
12. acetylcholinesterase
13. acetylcholine, norepinephrine
14. dura
15. subarachnoid
16. Meningitis
17. cauda equina
18. hemispheres
19. thalamus
20. hydrocephalus
21. frontal
22. Aphasia
23. Amnesia
24. antidiuretic hormone, oxytocin
25. dopamine
26. balance, coordination
27. brachial
28. nicotinic, muscarinic
29. Alzheimer's disease
30. Transient ischemic attacks (TIAs)

MATCHING

Group A

1. J	4. E	7. B	10. A
2. H	5. L	8. I	11. G
3. F	6. K	9. D	12. C

Group B

1. D	3. J	5. A	7. E	9. F
2. G	4. I	6. H	8. B	10. C

LABELING EXERCISE 8–1

1. F	4. B	6. C	8. D	10. E
2. A	5. G	7. I	9. K	11. J
3. H				

LABELING EXERCISE 8–2

1. J	5. P	9. K	13. A	16. M
2. N	6. B	10. F	14. L	17. O
3. D	7. R	11. Q	15. C	18. E
4. H	8. G	12. I		

LABELING EXERCISE 8–3

1. B	4. L	7. K	9. E	11. F
2. D	5. A	8. J	10. H	12. I
3. C	6. G			

SHORT ANSWER

1.
   a. *An action potential arrives at the synaptic knob.* The arriving action potential depolarizes the presynaptic membrane of the synaptic knob.
   b. *The neurotransmitter acetylcholine is released.* Depolarization of the presynaptic membrane causes the brief opening of calcium channels, which allows extracellular calcium ions to enter the synaptic knob. Their arrival triggers the exocytosis of the synaptic vesicles and the release of acetylcholine. The release of acetylcholine stops very soon thereafter because the calcium ions are rapidly removed from the cytoplasm by active transport mechanisms.
   c. *ACh binds and the postsynaptic membrane depolarizes.* The binding of acetylcholine to sodium channels causes them to open and allows sodium ions to enter. If the resulting depolarization of the postsynaptic membrane reaches threshold, an action potential is produced.
   d. *Acetylcholine is removed by acetylcholinesterase.* The effects on the postsynaptic membrane are temporary because the synaptic cleft and postsynaptic membrane contain the enzyme acetylcholinesterase. The acetylcholinesterase removes acetylcholine by breaking it into acetate and choline.

2. Excitatory neurotransmitters cause depolarization of the neuron. Acetylcholine and norepinephrine are examples of excitatory neurotransmitters. Inhibitory neurotransmitters cause hyperpolarization of the neuron. Dopamine, serotonin, and gamma-aminobutyric acid (GABA) are examples of inhibitory neurotransmitters.

3. The two divisions of the autonomic nervous system are the sympathetic and parasympathetic nervous systems. The sympathetic division is often called the "fight or flight" system because it usually stimulates tissue metabolism, increases alertness, and prepares the body to deal with emergencies. Examples of sympathetic nervous system or adrenergic receptors are alpha 1, alpha 2, beta 1, and beta 2 receptors.

The parasympathetic division of the ANS is often regarded as the "rest and repose" or "rest and digest" system because it conserves energy and promotes sedentary activities, such as digestion. Examples of parasympathetic or cholinergic receptors are muscarinic and nicotinic receptors.

4. The six major regions of the brain are the cerebrum, diencephalon, midbrain, pons, medulla oblongata, and the cerebellum.

5. A generalized tonic-clonic seizure is often referred to as a grand mal seizure. Grand mal seizures are the most familiar and dramatic seizure type. Grand mal seizures cause the patient to become stiff and fall to the ground. This is followed by alternating contraction and relaxation of the skeletal muscles. Urinary and fecal incontinence is common. This type of seizure usually lasts 6–90 seconds, and as it ends, the patient is left flaccid and unconscious. The patient may be confused for up to an hour following the attack (postictal confusion). Fatigue is common and may last for hours after the event.

Chapter 9

MULTIPLE CHOICE

1. D	10. B	19. D	28. B	37. B
2. C	11. D	20. B	29. B	38. C
3. E	12. C	21. B	30. C	39. B
4. D	13. B	22. A	31. B	40. C
5. C	14. D	23. E	32. C	41. C
6. D	15. B	24. B	33. C	42. D
7. A	16. D	25. D	34. B	43. A
8. A	17. B	26. C	35. D	44. C
9. A	18. C	27. C	36. B	45. C

ORDERING EXERCISE

1. D	3. F	5. E
2. A	4. B	6. C

FILL IN THE BLANK

1. Adaptation
2. referred pain
3. sigma
4. kappa
5. thermoreceptors
6. stretching, compression, twisting
7. touch, pressure, vibration
8. sty
9. inferior rectus, medial rectus, superior rectus, lateral rectus, inferior oblique, superior oblique
10. Ruffini
11. Baroreceptors
12. Chemoreceptors
13. olfactory
14. Umami
15. Schlemm
16. astigmatism
17. ciliary body
18. conjunctivitis or pink eye
19. sclera
20. anisocoria
21. rods, cones
22. fovea centralis
23. retina or neural tunic
24. blind spot
25. hyphema
26. cataract
27. accommodation
28. myopia
29. rhodopsin
30. A
31. tympanic
32. Dynamic
33. stapes
34. hair
35. Static
36. ampulla
37. presbyopia
38. presbycusis

39. macular degeneration
40. the thinning of mucous membranes

and a reduction in the number and sensitivity of taste buds

MATCHING

1. D	3. E	5. A	7. I	9. F
2. G	4. J	6. B	8. C	10. H

LABELING EXERCISE 9–1

1. D	5. O	9. F or B	13. P
2. B or F	6. G	10. K	14. M
3. E or L	7. J	11. A	15. N
4. H	8. I	12. C	16. E or L

LABELING EXERCISE 9–2

1. D	6. J	11. O	16. T	21. E
2. Q	7. U	12. Y	17. C	22. P
3. K	8. B	13. A	18. R	23. I
4. S	9. X	14. W	19. H	24. L
5. G	10. F	15. M	20. N	25. V

LABELING EXERCISE 9–3

1. F	4. E	7. N	10. A	13. G
2. M	5. J	8. H	11. K	14. D
3. B	6. C	9. L	12. I	

LABELING EXERCISE 9–4

1. A	4. I	7. D	10. L	12. M
2. H	5. C	8. K	11. F	13. G
3. B	6. J	9. E		

SHORT ANSWER

1. The first general sense receptor in the body is temperature. Within the dermis are thermoreceptors, which are nerve endings that sense a change in temperature. Although there are no structural differences between the two, the human body has three to four times more cold receptors than warm receptors.

   The second general sense receptor is pain. The pain receptors, or nociceptors, are also nerve endings that are found throughout the entire body. Depending on the type of pain, the nociceptors can send the pain impulse to myelinated nerve fibers that are responsible for transmitting fast or slow pain impulses.

   Touch, pressure, and positions are sensed by mechanoreceptors that are also found throughout the body. The three types of mechanoreceptors are: tactile receptors (touch), baroreceptors (pressure), and proprioceptors (position).

   The last general sense receptors are chemical receptors or chemoreceptors. These receptors are responsible for sensing changes in the chemical concentrations found in the body. Some examples of chemoreceptors are those in the carotid arteries and the aortic arch. These two receptors sense changes in pH, carbon dioxide levels, and oxygen concentrations in the arterial blood.

2. The four primary taste sensations are: sour, bitter, sweet, and salty.

3. The outermost layer is called the fibrous tunic. Within this section of the eye is the sclera and the cornea. The fibrous tunic provides mechanical support and some degree of physical protection of the eye, serves as an attachment site for extrinsic eye muscles, and assists in the focusing process.

The middle layer is called the vascular tunic. The vascular tunic contains all of the blood vessels, lymphatic tissues, and intrinsic eye muscles. Important functions include regulating the amount of light that enters the eye and controlling the shape of the lens.

The innermost layer is called the neural tunic, or retina. This portion of the eye contains the photoreceptors that respond to light.

4. Hyphema is blood in the anterior chamber of the eye. This sometimes can be seen by looking in the iris of the eye. The blood increases the pressure in the eye and can result in the loss of sight or function of the eye.

5. The pathophysiology of the pain response is very complex. There are both peripheral and central mediators of pain. The peripheral pain system is activated when nociceptors and free nerve endings register the original noxious stimulus in the peripheral tissues and transmit it to the central nervous system. Pain signals are integrated in the dorsal horn of the spinal cord. These are relayed to higher centers in the brain including the hypothalamus, thalamus, and the limbic and reticular activating systems. These centers integrate and process pain information, and allow the detection of and perception of pain. Interpretation, identification, and localization of pain also occur at these sites.

   Because pain is subjective, it is often difficult to assess. In the emergency setting, it is common to use a pain scale to determine the severity of a patient's pain. The most popular pain scale asks patients to rate their pain on a numeric scale that ranges from 0 to 10; 0 indicates no pain and 10 indicates the worst possible pain. Pain scale ratings can be monitored to determine the effectiveness of medications and other treatments.

   Analgesics are medications that help to alleviate pain. They may work on peripheral pain mediators, central pain mediators, or both. Nonsteroidal anti-inflammatory (NSAID) agents are commonly used for mild to moderate pain. NSAIDs primarily act on peripheral pain mediators and include aspirin, ibuprofen, naproxen, ketoprofen, and many others. These drugs decrease levels of inflammatory mediators, such as prostaglandins, generated at the site of tissue injury. Because they act peripherally, they do not cause sedation or respiratory depression and they do not interfere with bowel or bladder function. Acetaminophen (Tylenol) is also a peripherally acting analgesic. However, unlike the NSAIDs, it does not have anti-inflammatory properties and does not affect platelet aggregation (as does aspirin). Most peripherally acting analgesics must be administered orally or by topical application. The exception is ketorolac (Toradol), which is available for intramuscular or intravenous injection.

   Moderate to severe pain usually requires opioid analgesics. Opioid analgesics include morphine, codeine, hydromorphone, meperidine, fentanyl, and others. They are most effective when they are administered parenterally (outside of the digestive system). Common routes of opioid injection are subcutaneous, intramuscular, and intravenous.

Chapter 10

MULTIPLE CHOICE

1. D	11. C	21. B	31. C	41. C
2. B	12. D	22. A	32. D	42. C
3. B	13. B	23. B	33. C	43. A
4. D	14. A	24. C	34. C	44. C
5. A	15. B	25. B	35. A	45. B
6. B	16. C	26. A	36. B	46. B
7. C	17. D	27. A	37. D	47. C
8. B	18. B	28. B	38. A	48. B
9. D	19. D	29. D	39. D	49. A
10. D	20. D	30. C	40. B	50. A

FILL IN THE BLANK

1. Endocrine
2. hormone
3. Cyclic AMP (adenosine monophosphate)
4. infundibulum
5. regulatory hormones
6. ADH, oxytocin
7. sella turcica
8. Thyroid-stimulating
9. Follicle-stimulating
10. Growth
11. Gonadotropins
12. Melanocyte-stimulating
13. vasopressin
14. Diabetes insipidus
15. C
16. Graves'
17. Thyrotoxic
18. parathyroid hormone
19. Aldosterone
20. cortisol, corticosterone, cortisone
21. epinephrine, norepinephrine
22. insulin-dependent diabetes mellitus
23. Diabetic ketoacidosis
24. Renin
25. Angiotensin II
26. Atrial natriuretic peptide (ANP)
27. Resistin
28. epinephrine, norepinephrine
29. reproductive
30. diabetes, hypothyroidism

MATCHING

1. G	3. I	5. A	7. C	9. H
2. J	4. E	6. B	8. F	10. D

LABELING EXERCISE 10–1

1. D	4. I	6. K	8. J	10. G
2. F	5. B	7. H	9. C	11. E
3. A				

LABELING EXERCISE 10–2

Part I

1. H	3. A	5. C	7. G	8. E
2. F	4. D	6. B		

Part II

1. N	3. K	5. O	7. L	9. Q
2. J	4. I	6. M	8. P	

SHORT ANSWER

1. Excessive thirst and frequent urination can be caused by diabetes insipidus and diabetes mellitus.
2. Hormones or first messengers have no direct effect on the cell. They are typically too large to pass through the cell membrane. Hormones require a second messenger within the cell to trigger a certain response. The link between the first messenger and the second messenger usually involves a G protein, which is an enzyme complex that is coupled to a membrane receptor. The G protein is activated when a hormone binds to the hormone's receptor at the membrane surface. The second messenger may function as an enzyme activator or inhibitor, but the net result is a change in the cell's metabolic activities.
3. The seven hormones released by the anterior pituitary gland are the:
   thyroid-stimulating hormone, which triggers the release of thyroid hormones;
   adrenocorticotropic hormone, which stimulates the release of steroids from the adrenal cortex (the specific hormones are called glucocorticoids);
   follicle-stimulating hormone, which promotes egg development in females and sperm production in males;
   luteinizing hormone, which induces ovulation in females and stimulates the interstitial cells of the testes to produce sex hormones;
   prolactin, which stimulates mammary gland development and stimulates the production of milk by the mammary glands;
   growth hormone, which stimulates cell growth and cell replication by increasing the rate of protein synthesis; and
   melanocyte-stimulating hormone, which increases the production of melanin, the substance that helps control skin and hair pigmentation.
4. The following hormones are produced by the posterior pituitary gland:
   antidiuretic hormone (ADH), which is usually released as a response to a rise in the concentration of electrolytes in the blood. The primary function of ADH is to decrease the amount of water loss through the kidneys; and oxytocin, which stimulates smooth muscle contraction of the walls of the uterus during labor and delivery.
5. Cushing's syndrome, also called hyperadrenalism, is a common disorder most often seen in middle-age women. It results from an excessive amount of glucocorticoid release either from an abnormality of the anterior pituitary gland or the adrenal cortex.
   Addison's disease, also called adrenal insufficiency, occurs because of destruction of the adrenal cortex. This results in a decrease in glucocorticoid, mineralocorticoid, and androgen release.

Chapter 11

MULTIPLE CHOICE

1. D	10. A	19. C	28. C	37. C
2. D	11. B	20. A	29. C	38. A
3. C	12. B	21. D	30. C	39. C
4. C	13. B	22. A	31. D	40. C
5. D	14. B	23. A	32. C	41. B
6. B	15. B	24. C	33. D	42. D
7. B	16. D	25. A	34. C	43. B
8. B	17. C	26. B	35. B	44. D
9. B	18. C	27. C	36. C	45. C

FILL IN THE BLANK

1. Plasma
2. Red blood cells
3. White blood cells
4. Albumins
5. plasmin
6. intrinsic
7. hemocytoblasts or pluripotent stem cells
8. Red blood cells
9. Sickle cell disease
10. glucose
11. Anemia
12. Erythroblasts
13. increase cell division rates in erythroblasts, speed up maturation of red blood cells
14. hypoxia
15. B
16. agglutination
17. monocyte
18. Monocytes
19. lymphopoiesis
20. thrombocyte
21. 9–12 days
22. Hemostasis
23. Prothrombinase
24. heparin, Coumadin
25. stroke

MATCHING

1. I
2. G
3. A
4. E
5. B
6. J
7. C
8. F
9. D
10. H

LABELING EXERCISE 11–1

1. D   2. B   3. A   4. E   5. C

LABELING EXERCISE 11–2

1. I
2. K
3. M
4. H
5. G
6. A
7. F
8. D
9. L
10. J
11. B or N
12. C
13. E
14. B or N

SHORT ANSWER

1. The five primary functions of blood are:
   a. transporting dissolved gases, nutrients, hormones and metabolic wastes;
   b. regulating the pH and ion composition of interstitial fluids;
   c. restricting fluid losses at injury sites;
   d. defending against toxins and pathogens; and
   e. stabilizing body temperature.
2. The three classes of plasma proteins found in the blood are albumins, globulins, and fibrinogen.
3. *Neutrophils* comprise approximately 50 to 70 percent of all circulating white blood cells. A mature neutrophil has a very dense, contorted nucleus with two to five lobes that resemble beads on a string.

   Eosinophils are named so because their granules stain darkly with the red dye eosin. They usually represent 2–4 percent of circulating white blood cells (WBCs) and are similar in size to neutrophils.

   Basophils have numerous granules that stain darkly with basic dyes. In a standard blood smear, the granules are a deep purple or blue. These cells are somewhat smaller than neutrophils or eosinophils and are relatively rare; they account for less than 1 percent of the circulating WBC population.

   Monocytes are nearly twice the size of a typical erythrocyte. The nucleus is large and commonly oval or shaped like a kidney bean. Monocytes normally account for 2–8 percent of circulating WBCs.

   Lymphocytes are slightly larger than RBCs and contain a relatively large nucleus surrounded by a thin halo of cytoplasm. Lymphocytes account for 20–30 percent of the WBC population in blood.

4. Red blood cells (RBCs) contain the pigment hemoglobin, which binds and transports oxygen and carbon dioxide. Red blood cells are the most abundant of all blood cells; they account for 99.9 percent of the formed elements. The life span of a red blood cell is typically around 120 days long. Roughly one-third of the 75 trillion cells in the human body are red blood cells.

   White blood cells, also known as WBCs or leukocytes, can be distinguished from RBCs by their larger size and by the presence of a nucleus and other organelles. WBCs also lack hemoglobin. White blood cells help defend the body against invasion by pathogens, and they remove toxins, wastes, and abnormal or damaged cells.

5. Abnormal clot formation from a deep vein thrombosis or a pulmonary embolism can be a life-threatening situation. The process of dissolving a clot is called fibrinolysis. It begins with activation of the plasma protein plasminogen by tissue plasminogen activator (tPA). Damaged tissues release tPA. The activation of plasminogen produces the enzyme plasmin, which begins to digest the fibrin strands and thus erodes the clot foundation. Fibrinolytic agents cause the conversion of plasminogen to plasmin.

Chapter 12

MULTIPLE CHOICE

1. A	11. B	21. B	31. B	41. C
2. A	12. C	22. A	32. C	42. C
3. B	13. C	23. C	33. A	43. C
4. D	14. C	24. B	34. C	44. C
5. A	15. C	25. D	35. A	45. C
6. B	16. D	26. B	36. C	46. A
7. C	17. D	27. A	37. A	47. C
8. B	18. D	28. B	38. B	48. A
9. B	19. D	29. B	39. D	49. D
10. C	20. D	30. C	40. C	50. D

ORDERING EXERCISE

1. B   2. D   3. A   4. C   5. E

FILL IN THE BLANK

1. Arteries
2. Capillaries
3. pericardium/pericardial sac
4. anterior interventricular sulcus, posterior interventricular sulcus
5. epicardium
6. endocardium
7. Intercalated discs
8. vena cava
9. foramen ovale
10. Angina pectoris
11. aortic
12. abnormally long or short chordae tendinae, malfunctioning papillary muscles
13. aortic sinuses
14. right coronary
15. left coronary
16. myocardial infarction
17. atherosclerosis
18. ventricular tachycardia, ventricular fibrillation
19. ST elevation, new left bundle branch block
20. Percutaneous transluminal coronary angioplasty (PTCA)
21. Sodium
22. Tachycardia
23. internal automatic cardioverter-defibrillator (IACD)

24. cardiac output
25. stroke volume
26. commotio cordis
27. Frank-Starling principle
28. Valvular heart disease
29. Coronary Artery Bypass Graft (CABG)
30. hyperkalemia

MATCHING

1. D	3. A	5. J	7. C	9. H
2. F	4. G	6. B	8. E	10. I

LABELING EXERCISE 12–1

1. E	3. G	5. H	7. F
2. B	4. A	6. D	8. C

LABELING EXERCISE 12–2

1. G	3. F	5. B	7. H	9. D
2. I	4. C	6. J	8. A	10. E

LABELING EXERCISE 12–3

1. L	6. P	10. K	14. G	18. I
2. F	7. H	11. T	15. S	19. O
3. J	8. R	12. B	16. A	20. E
4. N	9. C	13. U	17. Q	21. M
5. D				

LABELING EXERCISE 12–4

1. B	3. D	5. C	7. A
2. H	4. G	6. F	8. E

LABELING EXERCISE 12–5

1. H	4. D	6. K	8. E	10. C
2. F	5. B	7. A	9. I	11. G
3. J				

LABELING EXERCISE 12–6

1. F	3. G	5. H	7. I	9. J
2. A	4. B	6. C	8. D	10. E

LABELING EXERCISE 12–7

1. B	2. D	3. C	4. E	5. A

SHORT ANSWER

1. From the right atrium, the unoxygenated blood travels through the tricuspid valve to the right ventricle. From the right ventricle the blood travels through the semilunar pulmonic valve into the pulmonary artery and into the pulmonary circulation. At this point the blood moves through the pulmonary capillary system and becomes oxygenated. The blood then travels to the left atria via the pulmonary veins. From the left atria the blood travels through the mitral valve into the left ventricle. Blood then moves from the left ventricle through the aortic valve into the aorta. The aorta then moves the oxygenated blood into the systemic circulation. The blood moves through the systemic circulation back to the right atrium.

2. SA node, intranodal pathways, AV node, bundle of His, left and right bundle branches, Purkinje fibers

3. The signs and symptoms of acute coronary syndrome include chest pain, difficulty breathing, sweating (diaphoresis), nausea, vomiting, and dizziness.

Half of all patients who die during an acute coronary syndrome do so because of a disruption in the cardiac conduction system called a dysrhythmia. Common dysrhythmias associated with myocardial ischemia and sudden death are ventricular fibrillation or ventricular tachycardia. In ventricular fibrillation, no organized electrical activity occurs, and the myocardial muscle mass simply quivers, or fibrillates. Thus, no myocardial contraction takes place. Ventricular fibrillation can be effectively treated by defibrillation, which is the rapid application of an electrical countershock. Defibrillation stops the irregular electrical activity of the heart, which allows the normal pacemaker of the heart to resume control.

4. The first phase is rapid depolarization of the cell. At threshold, voltage-regulated sodium channels open, and the influx of sodium ions rapidly depolarizes the sarcolemma. The sodium channels close when the transmembrane potential reaches +30 mV.

The second phase is the plateau phase. As the cell now begins to actively pump sodium ions out, voltage-regulated calcium channels open and extracellular calcium ions enter the sarcoplasm. The calcium channels remain open for a relatively long period, and the entering positive charges (Ca^{2+}) roughly balance the loss of Na^+ from the cell. The increased concentration of calcium within the cell also triggers the release of Ca^{2+} from reserves in the sarcoplasmic reticulum (SR), which continue the contraction.

The third phase is repolarization. As the calcium channels begin to close, potassium channels open and potassium ions (K+) rush out of the cell. The net result is a repolarization that restores the resting potential.

5. The sympathetic release of NE at synapses in the myocardium and the release of NE and E by the adrenal medullae stimulate cardiac muscle cell metabolism and increase the force and degree of contraction. The result is an increase in stroke volume.

The primary effect of parasympathetic ACh release is inhibition, which results in a decrease in the force of cardiac contractions. Because parasympathetic innervation of the ventricles is relatively limited, the greatest reduction in contractile force occurs in the atria.

Chapter 13

MULTIPLE CHOICE

1. B	11. A	21. C	31. D	41. C
2. A	12. D	22. C	32. D	42. D
3. B	13. C	23. C	33. C	43. B
4. B	14. C	24. D	34. B	44. C
5. D	15. C	25. D	35. C	45. D
6. B	16. B	26. D	36. B	46. B
7. C	17. A	27. B	37. D	47. C
8. B	18. A	28. B	38. A	48. C
9. C	19. C	29. B	39. C	49. D
10. C	20. C	30. D	40. D	50. B

FILL IN THE BLANK

1. venules
2. sphygmomanometer
3. Edema
4. arteriosclerosis
5. anastomosis
6. valves
7. peripheral resistance
8. Viscosity
9. Anemia
10. 120, 2
11. precapillary sphincter
12. hypertension
13. cardiac output, peripheral vascular resistance
14. cardiac output, peripheral vascular resistance, blood pressure
15. vasodilators
16. aortic, carotid
17. epinephrine, norepinephrine
18. Antidiuretic hormone
19. Angiotensin II
20. kidneys
21. Atrial natriuretic peptide
22. Shock (hypoperfusion)
23. Acute pulmonary embolism
24. pulmonary veins
25. aneurysm
26. right subclavian artery, right common carotid artery
27. radial, ulnar
28. circle of Willis
29. phrenic
30. Raynaud's phenomenon
31. ductus venosus
32. foramen ovale
33. ductus arteriosus
34. pulmonary embolism
35. 85–95

MATCHING

1. G	3. A	5. H	7. B	9. E
2. I	4. C	6. J	8. D	10. F

LABELING EXERCISE 13–1

1. P	7. V	13. D	19. M	25. U
2. C	8. E	14. A	20. AA	26. S
3. R	9. X	15. L	21. G	27. B
4. N	10. Z	16. W	22. I	28. Q
5. F	11. J	17. DD	23. Y	29. O
6. T	12. BB	18. CC	24. K	30. H

LABELING EXERCISE 13–2

1. R	8. P	15. V	22. B	29. Q
2. N	9. D	16. HH	23. II	30. AA
3. G	10. I	17. A	24. L	31. U
4. Y	11. C	18. Z	25. EE	32. X
5. E	12. W	19. K	26. GG	33. H
6. BB	13. FF	20. O	27. F	34. CC
7. DD	14. M	21. T	28. J	35. S

LABELING EXERCISE 13–3

1. F	3. I or A	5. D	7. B	9. C
2. J	4. A or I	6. H	8. G	10. E

LABELING EXERCISE 13–4

1. R	7. G	13. L	19. Z	24. K
2. N	8. V	14. F	20. E	25. C
3. I	9. Y	15. P	21. X	26. S
4. T	10. B	16. BB	22. H	27. M
5. D	11. AA	17. A	23. U	28. Q
6. W	12. J	18. O		

SHORT ANSWER

1. The first source is vascular resistance. Most of the vascular resistance occurs in the arterioles, which are extremely muscular. The walls of an arteriole with a 30-μm internal diameter, for example, can have a 20-μm-thick layer of smooth muscle. Local, neural, and hormonal stimuli that stimulate or inhibit this smooth muscle tissue can adjust the diameters of these vessels, and a small change in diameter can produce a very large change in resistance.

   The second source is viscosity. The property called viscosity is the resistance to flow that results from interactions among molecules and suspended materials in a liquid. Liquids of low viscosity, such as water, flow at low pressures; whereas thick, syrupy liquids such as molasses flow only under higher pressures. Because whole blood contains plasma proteins and suspended blood cells, it has a viscosity about five times that of water.

   The last source is turbulence. Turbulence is responsible for increasing resistance in the arteries. Turbulence normally occurs when blood flows between the heart's chambers and from the heart into the aorta and pulmonary trunk. In addition to increasing resistance, turbulence generates the third and fourth heart sounds often heard through a stethoscope. Turbulent blood flow across damaged or misaligned heart valves produces the sound of heart murmurs.

2. Atherosclerosis is the formation of lipid deposits in the tunica media of the artery that is associated with damage to the endothelial lining. Atherosclerosis tends to develop in individuals whose blood contains elevated levels of plasma lipids, specifically cholesterol. Circulating cholesterol is transported to peripheral tissues in protein–lipid complexes called lipoproteins.

   When cholesterol-rich lipoproteins remain in circulation for an extended period, circulating monocytes begin removing them from the bloodstream. Eventually the monocytes, which are now filled with lipid droplets, attach themselves to the endothelia of blood vessels. These cells then release growth factors that stimulate the divisions of smooth muscle cells near the tunica interna. The vessel wall thickens with plaque made from fat cells, smooth muscle cells, and monocytes.

3. Arteriosclerosis is a thickening and toughening of arterial walls. Arteriosclerosis of coronary vessels is responsible for coronary artery disease (CAD), and arteriosclerosis of arteries that supply the brain can lead to strokes. The two major forms of arteriosclerosis are focal calcification and atherosclerosis. In focal calcification, degenerating smooth muscle in the tunica media is replaced by calcium deposits. It occurs as part of the aging process and is associated with atherosclerosis. Reference the answer to question #2 for a description of atherosclerosis.

4. An aneurysm is a bulging in the weakened wall of a blood vessel. Aneurysms are at risk for rupture. Most aneurysms result from atherosclerosis and involve the aorta because the blood pressure there is higher than at any other vessel in the body. An aneurysm usually occurs gradually. Eventually, blood surges into the aortic wall through a tear in the aortic tunica intima. Aortic aneurysms can occur in the chest or abdomen. Thoracic aortic

©2008 Pearson Education, Inc.
Anatomy & Physiology for Emergency Care, 2nd ed.

aneurysms usually involve the arch of the aorta. Rupture of a thoracic aortic aneurysm is usually a catastrophic event.

5. Renin starts a chain reaction that ultimately converts an inactive plasma protein, angiotensinogen, to the hormone angiotensin II. Angiotensin II stimulates cardiac output and triggers arteriole constriction, which in turn elevates systemic blood pressure almost immediately. As the levels of renin go up, so do the levels of angiotensin II.

Chapter 14

MULTIPLE CHOICE

1. D	11. C	21. B	31. C	41. D
2. D	12. D	22. C	32. B	42. A
3. D	13. A	23. A	33. B	43. B
4. C	14. D	24. B	34. A	44. C
5. B	15. C	25. D	35. D	45. C
6. D	16. B	26. D	36. D	46. D
7. B	17. D	27. D	37. C	47. D
8. B	18. A	28. B	38. A	48. B
9. C	19. C	29. C	39. B	49. C
10. D	20. B	30. D	40. D	50. D

FILL IN THE BLANK

1. Immunity
2. Pathogens
3. thoracic duct
4. Lymphocytes
5. T cells
6. Suppressor T cells
7. B cells
8. lymphopoiesis
9. hemocytoblasts
10. thymus
11. Thymosins
12. Nonspecific
13. Specific
14. phagocytes
15. neutralization
16. Interferons
17. temporary repair of the injured site, slowing the spread of pathogens, mobilizing a wide range of defenses
18. Necrosis
19. tonsils
20. perforins
21. Active
22. naturally acquired passive
23. antigen-presenting cells (APCs)
24. Helper T
25. Suppressor T
26. IgM
27. IgE
28. IgM
29. RNA
30. Tumor necrosis factors
31. Y
32. Delayed
33. Immediate
34. allergic reaction
35. insect bites
36. Autoimmune disorders
37. antigens
38. broncho-constriction, contraction of the intestines
39. urticaria (hives)
40. epinephrine

MATCHING

1. F	3. G	5. H	7. C	9. E
2. I	4. B	6. A	8. J	10. D

LABELING EXERCISE 14–1

1. F	4. C	7. N	10. G	13. E
2. J	5. L	8. D	11. A	14. K
3. I	6. H	9. O	12. M	15. B

LABELING EXERCISE 14–2

1. A	3. D	5. F	7. E
2. C	4. H	6. G	8. B

SHORT ANSWER

1. Active immunity appears after exposure to an antigen as a consequence of the immune response. Even though the immune system is capable of defending against an enormous number of antigens, the appropriate defenses are mobilized only after an individual's lymphocytes encounter a particular antigen. Active immunity may develop as a result of natural exposure to an antigen in the environment (naturally acquired active immunity) or from deliberate exposure to an antigen (induced active immunity).

   Passive immunity is produced by the transfer of antibodies to an individual from some other source. Naturally acquired passive immunity results when antibodies produced by a mother protect her baby against infections during gestation (by crossing the placenta) or in early infancy (through breast milk). In induced passive immunity, antibodies are administered to fight infection or prevent disease after exposure to the pathogen.

2. All T cells originate within the thymus gland. The four types of T cells are cytotoxic T cells, helper T cells, memory T cells, and suppressor T cells.

3. The three main functions of the lymphatic system are the production, maintenance, and distribution of lymphocytes; the return of fluid and solutes from peripheral tissues to the blood; and the distribution of hormones, nutrients, and waste products from their tissues of origin to the general circulation.

4. B cells originate in the bone marrow. B cells can differentiate into plasma cells, which produce and secrete antibodies—soluble proteins that are also called immunoglobulins. Antibodies bind to specific chemical targets called antigens, which are usually pathogens, parts or products of pathogens, or other foreign compounds. B cells are responsible for antibody-mediated immunity.

5. Nonspecific defenses do not distinguish between one threat and another. These defenses, which are present at birth, include physical barriers, phagocytic cells, immunological surveillance, interferons, complement, inflammation, and fever. They provide the body with a defensive capability known as nonspecific resistance.

   Specific defenses protect against particular threats. Many specific defenses develop after birth as a result of exposure to environmental hazards or infectious agents. Specific defenses are dependent on the activities of lymphocytes.

Chapter 15

MULTIPLE CHOICE

1. D	11. A	21. C	31. B	41. B
2. C	12. B	22. D	32. B	42. B
3. D	13. B	23. B	33. C	43. C
4. B	14. B	24. A	34. D	44. B
5. B	15. A	25. A	35. B	45. B
6. C	16. B	26. A	36. C	46. D
7. D	17. C	27. A	37. C	47. C
8. C	18. B	28. C	38. C	48. A
9. C	19. D	29. B	39. C	49. B
10. D	20. B	30. C	40. C	50. B

FILL IN THE BLANK

1. external nares
2. End-tidal carbon dioxide (ETCO$_2$)
3. glottis
4. epiglottis
5. Adam's apple
6. tracheal cartilages
7. secondary bronchi
8. constriction
9. alveolar ducts
10. Sudden infant death syndrome (SIDS)
11. pleura
12. hemothorax
13. Anoxia
14. Positive-end expiratory pressure (PEEP)
15. tidal volume
16. expiratory reserve volume
17. 20.9 percent
18. Emphysema
19. Asthma
20. 98
21. 80
22. bicarbonate ions
23. increase
24. decrease
25. inflation reflex

MATCHING

1. E	3. H	5. B	7. C	9. J
2. D	4. A	6. I	8. F	10. G

LABELING EXERCISE 15–1

1. G	5. P	9. R	13. J	17. E
2. I	6. L	10. A	14. Q	18. M
3. N	7. B	11. S	15. C	19. H
4. D	8. K	12. F	16. O	

LABELING EXERCISE 15–2

1. O	6. F	11. W	16. X	21. R
2. D	7. U	12. H	17. I	22. G
3. Q	8. L	13. N	18. K	23. M
4. J	9. Y	14. V	19. T	24. P
5. S	10. B	15. E	20. A	25. C

LABELING EXERCISE 15–3

1. C	3. F	5. D	7. B
2. E	4. A	6. G	

SHORT ANSWER

1. The five functions of the respiratory system are:
   a. providing a large area for gas exchange between air and circulating blood;
   b. protecting the respiratory surfaces from dehydration and temperature changes and defending against invading pathogens;
   c. moving air to and from the gas-exchange surfaces of the lungs;
   d. producing sounds that permit speech, singing, and nonverbal auditory communication; and
   e. providing olfactory sensations to the central nervous system for the sense of smell.

2. Asthma is a chronic inflammatory disorder of the airways. The widespread inflammation of the airways leads to an obstruction of airflow. The factors that are known to bring on an asthma attack are often called triggers. Some common triggers are: allergens, cold air, exercise, foods, stress, and certain medications.

3. Vital capacity is the maximum amount of air that can be moved into and out of the respiratory system in a single respiration. It is calculated by adding together the inspiratory reserve, expiratory reserve, and the tidal volumes.

4. The three methods by which the body transports carbon dioxide in the blood are: dissolved in plasma; bound to hemoglobin within the red blood cell; converted to carbonic acid (H$_2$CO$_3$).

5. Emphysema results from a destruction of the alveolar walls distal to the terminal bronchioles. Emphysema also causes a weakening of the walls of small bronchioles. When the walls are destroyed, the lungs lose their capacity to recoil and air remains trapped in the bronchioles. Residual volume increases due to the trapped air, but the vital capacity remains the same. This increase in pressure destroys the lung tissue, which leads to further alveolar collapse. The major contributor to emphysema is cigarette smoking.

Chapter 16

MULTIPLE CHOICE

1. B	11. D	21. B	31. C	41. D
2. D	12. D	22. A	32. C	42. B
3. B	13. D	23. C	33. C	43. C
4. B	14. A	24. C	34. D	44. B
5. A	15. B	25. C	35. B	45. A
6. C	16. C	26. B	36. D	46. B
7. B	17. D	27. C	37. C	47. B
8. D	18. B	28. C	38. B	48. C
9. B	19. C	29. A	39. B	49. B
10. D	20. B	30. C	40. D	50. C

FILL IN THE BLANK

1. mucosa
2. submucosa
3. peristalsis
4. segmentation
5. Salivary amylase
6. dentin
7. pharynx
8. esophagus
9. deglutition
10. esophagitis
11. chyme
12. Ascites
13. Gastroenteritis
14. simple columnar
15. 1500 mL
16. intrinsic factor, hydrochloric acid
17. rennin
18. gastric ulcers
19. intestinal
20. small intestine
21. plicae
22. Serotonin
23. Secretin
24. Gastric inhibitory peptide
25. Gastrin
26. cholecystokinin
27. falciform ligament
28. Kupffer cells
29. emulsification
30. Hepatitis C
31. bile storage
32. right upper quadrant
33. lymphatic
34. haustra
35. taeniae coli
36. prothrombin
37. hydrolysis
38. B$_1$
39. constipation
40. Cirrhosis

MATCHING

1. F	3. A	5. B	7. C	9. G
2. E	4. H	6. I	8. J	10. D

LABELING EXERCISE 16–1

1. I	3. F	5. A	7. B	9. G
2. C	4. H	6. D	8. J	10. E

LABELING EXERCISE 16–2

1. C	3. A	5. D	6. F	7. B
2. E	4. G			

LABELING EXERCISE 16–3

1. O	5. I	9. N	13. J
2. K	6. H	10. A	14. D or P
3. G	7. E	11. L	15. C
4. B	8. P or D	12. F	16. M

LABELING EXERCISE 16–4

1. C	3. G	5. F	7. I	9. H
2. E	4. A	6. J	8. D	10. B

LABELING EXERCISE 16–5

1. K	6. O	11. I	16. G	21. N
2. M	7. A	12. E	17. P	22. H
3. C	8. S	13. R	18. X	23. L
4. T	9. U	14. J	19. D	24. B
5. Q	10. W	15. V	20. F	

SHORT ANSWER

1. Parietal cells secrete intrinsic factor and hydrochloric acid. The intrinsic factor facilitates the absorption of vitamin B_{12} into the intestine. Hydrochloric acid lowers the pH of the gastric juice, which keeps the pH of stomach contents between 1.5 and 2.0. This acidity helps kill bacteria, break down plant cell walls and connective tissues found in meat, and activate the pepsinogen that is released from the chief cells.

   Chief cells secrete a protein called pepsinogen. When pepsinogen comes in contact with the hydrochloric acid, the acidity converts the pepsinogen into the proteolytic enzyme pepsin.

2. The four intestinal hormones are gastrin, secretin, cholecystokinin, and gastric inhibitory peptide. Gastrin aids in digestion by breaking down proteins and stimulates the production of acids and enzymes. Secretin increases the secretion of bile and buffers by the pancreas and liver. Cholecystokinin accelerates the production and secretion of all types of digestive enzymes and causes the gallbladder to release stored bile into the duodenum. Gastric inhibitory peptide (GIP) inhibits gastric activity and stimulates the release of insulin from the pancreatic islets.

3. The majority of peptic ulcers are caused by either nonsteroidal anti-inflammatory medications, acid-stimulating products like alcohol or nicotine, or by the bacteria *Helicobacter pylori*. The first two are fairly easy to treat because the patients are told to discontinue taking the medications and acid-stimulating products and the symptoms usually go away. New research has shown that over 80 percent of all peptic ulcers are actually caused by the bacteria *Helicobacter pylori*. Patients are put on antacids and antibiotics are administered to kill the bacteria rather than merely treat the patient's symptoms.

4. Mallory-Weiss syndrome is an esophageal laceration most often seen from alcoholic liver damage. The damage to the esophagus is usually caused secondary to vomiting. If not treated, life-threatening or difficult-to-control hemorrhage can result.

5. The three phases involved in gastric secretion are the cephalic, gastric, and intestinal phases.

Chapter 17

MULTIPLE CHOICE

1. C	5. C	9. C	13. B	17. B
2. B	6. B	10. A	14. C	18. D
3. C	7. D	11. D	15. C	19. C
4. D	8. B	12. D	16. B	20. C

21. B	26. B	31. A	36. C	41. D
22. C	27. D	32. D	37. D	42. C
23. B	28. C	33. C	38. C	43. B
24. A	29. D	34. C	39. D	44. D
25. A	30. D	35. B	40. B	45. D

FILL IN THE BLANK

1. lipids
2. Coenzymes
3. oxygen
4. cellular respiration
5. NAD
6. chemiosmosis
7. ATP synthase
8. carbon dioxide
9. lipogenesis
10. good cholesterol
11. vitamin B_6
12. chylomicrons
13. Deamination
14. ketone bodies
15. ketosis
16. hyperglycemia
17. 200 mg/dL
18. Minerals
19. Wernicke's encephalopathy, Korsakoff's syndrome
20. radiation

MATCHING

1. E	3. H	5. I	7. B	9. D
2. G	4. A	6. J	8. C	10. F

LABELING EXERCISE 17–1

1. E, F, H, *or* J	5. E, F, H, *or* J	9. E, F, H, *or* J
2. A	6. C	10. E, F, H, *or* J
3. G	7. I	11. K
4. B	8. D	

SHORT ANSWER

1. Glycolysis is the breakdown of glucose into pyruvic acid. The main function of glycolysis is to generate the pyruvic acid that then enters the tricarboxylic acid (TCA) cycle. Glycolysis does not require oxygen for this breakdown to occur, and it generates a net gain of two ATP molecules during this process.

   The TCA cycle requires oxygen and is responsible for the removal of hydrogen atoms by the coenzymes nicotinamide adenine dinucleotide (NAD) and flavine adenine dinucleotide (FAD). These two coenzymes form NADH and $FADH_2$ and transfer the hydrogen atoms to the electron transport system (ETS), which is the most important mechanism for the generation of ATP.

2. Cellular respiration is the mitochondrial activity responsible for the production of ATP.

3. A lack of oxygen is referred to as hypoxia. Since oxygen is essential for the mitochondria to produce ATP, hypoxia inhibits or stops the TCA cycle and the electron transport system, which thereby stops the mitochondria from producing the 32 molecules of ATP it normally would.

4. Deamination prepares an amino acid for breakdown in the TCA cycle. Deamination removes an amino group that then generates an ammonia molecule.

   Transamination is the creation of a new amino acid by attaching the amino group of an amino acid to another carbon chain. Transamination enables cells to synthesize new amino acids needed for protein synthesis.

5. Hypoglycemia is an inadequate amount of available glucose for the cells; whereas hyperglycemia is an excessive amount of available glucose.

Chapter 18

MULTIPLE CHOICE

1. D	12. D	23. C	34. C	45. B
2. B	13. C	24. A	35. C	46. C
3. B	14. B	25. D	36. D	47. A
4. C	15. B	26. B	37. B	48. C
5. A	16. A	27. C	38. C	49. A
6. B	17. B	28. A	39. B	50. B
7. D	18. D	29. B	40. C	51. C
8. B	19. B	30. B	41. B	52. A
9. B	20. D	31. E	42. A	53. D
10. D	21. B	32. C	43. C	54. A
11. B	22. C	33. C	44. C	55. D

FILL IN THE BLANK

1. urinary system
2. urine
3. cortex and pyramids
4. afferent arteriole
5. Uric acid
6. podocytes
7. Incontinence
8. Creatine phosphate
9. 60 to 70
10. aldosterone
11. sympathetic
12. Respiratory acidosis
13. renin-angiotensin
14. ureters
15. kidney stone or renal calculus

ORDERING EXERCISE

1. C	3. F	5. D
2. E	4. A	6. B

MATCHING

1. D	3. H	5. J	7. C	9. I
2. E	4. A	6. B	8. F	10. G

LABELING EXERCISE 18–1

1. I	4. K	7. G	9. J	11. H
2. B	5. F	8. A	10. C	12. E
3. D	6. L			

LABELING EXERCISE 18–2

1. C	3. A	5. B	7. I	9. E
2. F	4. D	6. G	8. H	

LABELING EXERCISE 18–3

1. B	4. A	7. E	9. C	11. F
2. K	5. D	8. J	10. L	12. I
3. H	6. G			

LABELING EXERCISE 18–4

1. C	4. L	7. G	10. J	12. H
2. I	5. A	8. D	11. B	13. F
3. E	6. M	9. K		

LABELING EXERCISE 18–5

1. B	3. G	5. C	7. F	9. A
2. E	4. I	6. D	8. H	

SHORT ANSWER

1. Hemodialysis is the most common type of dialysis used to treat acute renal failure. The patient is attached to a machine in which his blood comes in contact with a large semipermeable membrane. On the opposite side of the semipermeable membrane is a specialized dialysate solution that is hypo-osmolar for substances that must be removed from the blood. Blood contacts this membrane, and targeted substances diffuse into the dialysate. The net effect of dialysis is the correction of electrolyte abnormalities and blood volume and the removal of toxic substances such as urea or creatinine. For patients who require chronic hemodialysis, a vascular shunt, which is capable of handling blood flow of 300–400 mL per minute, is placed between a suitable vein and artery for dialysis access.

2. The actions of atrial natriuretic peptide (ANP) oppose the effects of the renin-angiotensin system. It is released by atrial cardiac muscle cells when blood volume and blood pressure are too high. ANP decreases the rate of sodium ion reabsorption in the distal convoluted tubule, which results in increased sodium ion loss in the urine. ANP also dilates the glomerular capillaries, which results in increased glomerular filtration and urinary water loss; and inactivates the renin-angiotensin system through the inhibition of renin, aldosterone, and antidiuretic hormone (ADH) secretion. The net result is an accelerated loss of sodium ions and an increase in the volume of urine produced. This combination lowers blood volume and blood pressure.

3. The major sign or symptom of kidney stones is pain. Typically, the patient first notes discomfort as a vague, visceral pain in one flank. Within 30 to 60 minutes it progresses to an extremely sharp pain that may remain in the flank or migrate downward and anteriorly toward the groin. As a rule, patients with kidney stones cannot lay still. They continuously move or pace due to the unrelenting nature of the pain. Stones that lodge in the lowest part of the ureter, within the bladder wall, often cause characteristic bladder symptoms such as frequency during the day or during the night (nocturia), urgency, and painful urination.

4. In metabolic acidosis, there is an accumulation of noncarbonic acids or a loss of bicarbonate. Causes include lactic acidosis (from poor perfusion), renal failure, or diabetic ketoacidosis. The buffer systems attempt to compensate. Respirations are increased as the pH falls, which results in elimination of CO_2. The renal system secretes excess hydrogen ions.

   Metabolic alkalosis is due to an increase in bicarbonate or to excessive loss of metabolic acids. Causes include prolonged vomiting, gastrointestinal suctioning, excessive bicarbonate intake, or diuretic therapy. Vomiting and gastrointestinal suctioning can cause loss of gastric acids, which ultimately leads to metabolic alkalosis.

5. The five age-related changes that occur to the urinary system in the elderly are:
   a. a decline in the number of functional nephrons;
   b. a reduction in the glomerular filtration rate (GFR);
   c. a reduced sensitivity to antidiuretic hormone (ADH) and aldosterone;
   d. problems with the micturition reflex; and
   e. a decrease in total body water content.

Chapter 19

MULTIPLE CHOICE

1. C	11. B	21. D	31. B	41. C
2. D	12. C	22. C	32. B	42. D
3. C	13. B	23. A	33. D	43. D
4. C	14. D	24. C	34. B	44. A
5. C	15. B	25. C	35. C	45. C
6. B	16. C	26. A	36. C	46. D
7. B	17. B	27. B	37. D	47. D
8. C	18. B	28. C	38. A	48. B
9. C	19. D	29. D	39. C	49. D
10. A	20. D	30. A	40. C	50. C

FILL IN THE BLANK

1. testes
2. cryptorchidism
3. Testicular torsion
4. Mitosis
5. tetrad
6. haploid
7. capacitation
8. foreskin or prepuce
9. interstitial cell-stimulating hormone
10. Mittelschmerz
11. dyspareunia
12. infundibulum
13. corpus luteum
14. cervix
15. Peg
16. Endometriosis
17. pelvic inflammatory disease (PID)
18. gonorrhea, chlamydia
19. vulva
20. Infertility

MATCHING

1. E	3. H	5. B	7. C	9. G
2. F	4. A	6. J	8. D	10. I

LABELING EXERCISE 19–1

1. C	4. M	7. N	10. F	13. J
2. K	5. H	8. I	11. L	14. G
3. E	6. D	9. A	12. B	

LABELING EXERCISE 19–2

1. B	3. C	5. A	6. F	7. G
2. E	4. D			

LABELING EXERCISE 19–3

1. J	5. D	8. P	11. H	14. M
2. G	6. N	9. I	12. O	15. C
3. L	7. F	10. A	13. E	16. K
4. B				

LABELING EXERCISE 19–4

1. C	5. M	9. R	13. D	16. E
2. K	6. B	10. A	14. N	17. L
3. I	7. P	11. O	15. J	18. G
4. F	8. H	12. Q		

SHORT ANSWER

1. Priapism is a prolonged, usually painful, penile erection that is not associated with sexual arousal. It is associated with sickle cell disease, spinal cord injury, spinal anesthesia, leukemia, and drugs.
2. When an egg is released from the ovary, a corpus luteum cyst is often left in its place. Occasionally, cysts develop independent of ovulation. When a cyst ruptures, a small amount of blood spills into the abdomen, which can cause abdominal pain and rebound tenderness. A patient with a ruptured cyst is likely to complain of moderate to severe unilateral abdominal pain, which may radiate to her back.
3. Sexually transmitted diseases (STDs) are infections contracted by intimate or sexual contact. In the United States, the most common STDs are chlamydia, gonorrhea, syphilis, genital warts, and herpes simplex virus, type 2.
4. Combination birth control pills can worsen problems associated with severe hypertension, diabetes mellitus, epilepsy, gallbladder disease, heart trouble, and acne. They can also increase the risk for venous thrombosis, strokes, pulmonary embolism, and (for women over 35) heart disease.
5. Testicular torsion usually compromises blood supply to the testicle and results in severe scrotal and abdominal pain. If emergency surgery is not performed within six hours, the testicle may be lost.

Chapter 20

MULTIPLE CHOICE

1. C	8. D	15. B	22. B	29. C
2. A	9. C	16. C	23. B	30. C
3. C	10. C	17. D	24. A	31. C
4. A	11. D	18. D	25. D	32. B
5. C	12. A	19. B	26. D	33. B
6. B	13. B	20. D	27. C	34. D
7. D	14. C	21. C	28. B	35. C

FILL IN THE BLANK

1. Hyaluronidase
2. Polyspermy
3. amphimixis
4. Cleavage
5. Ectopic pregnancy
6. placenta
7. yolk sac
8. episiotomy
9. cesarean section
10. conjoined or Siamese twins
11. colostrum
12. miscarriage
13. complete abortion
14. therapeutic abortion
15. alleles
16. Cystic fibrosis
17. Trisomy 21 or Down syndrome
18. Klinefelter syndrome
19. Trauma
20. Abruptio placentae

MATCHING

1. D	3. F	5. A	7. C	9. G
2. H	4. J	6. B	8. E	10. I

LABELING EXERCISE 20–1

1. G	4. B	7. J	10. E
2. A	5. I	8. D	11. L
3. H	6. C	9. K	12. F

LABELING EXERCISE 20–2

1. I	4. K	7. O	10. N	13. J
2. A or F	5. M	8. G	11. L	14. H
3. D	6. B	9. A or F	12. E	15. C

SHORT ANSWER

1. Ectopic pregnancy most often presents as abdominal pain, which starts as diffuse tenderness and then localizes as a sharp pain in the lower abdominal quadrant on the affected side. This pain is due to rupture of the fallopian tube when the fetus outgrows the available space. The ruptured fallopian tube also causes intra-abdominal bleeding. As this bleeding continues, the abdomen becomes rigid and the pain intensifies and is often referred to the shoulder on

the affected side. The pain is often accompanied by syncope, vaginal bleeding, and shock. The woman also may report that she missed a period or that her last menstrual period (LMP) occurred 4 to 6 weeks ago.

2. Gravidity 3, parity 2 (G₃P₂)
3. Cystic fibrosis is an autosomal recessive disease that affects the exocrine glands. The two organs that are impacted the most are the lungs and pancreas.
4. Patients with sickle cell disease are often frequent visitors to hospital emergency departments, as they periodically develop sickle cell crisis, in which blood flow to small blood vessels in organs such as the bones and spleen become occluded. Sickle cell crisis can be extremely painful, requiring high doses of narcotics to achieve pain control.
5. The uterus of a supine patient in late pregnancy may compress the inferior vena cava and reduce the venous return to the heart. This may induce hypotension in the uninjured patient and have severe consequences in the hemorrhaging trauma patient.

Comprehensive Exam Answer Key

MULTIPLE CHOICE

1. B	36. A	68. C
2. D	37. C	69. A
3. D	38. C	70. D
4. D	39. B	71. C
5. B	40. D	72. B
6. C	41. C	73. A
7. C	42. C	74. D
8. D	43. B	75. D
9. B	44. D	76. C
10. A	45. A	77. B
11. A	46. D	78. B
12. C	47. C	79. B
13. D	48. B	80. B
14. D	49. B	81. C
15. C	50. C	82. C
16. A	51. D	83. B
17. B	52. B	84. D
18. B	53. A	85. C
19. C	54. C	86. D
20. B	55. C	87. D
21. C	56. D	88. D
22. C	57. A	89. C
23. D	58. B	90. C
24. C	59. A	91. C
25. C	60. A	92. C
26. B	61. D	93. B
27. C	62. D	94. B
28. B	63. C	95. C
29. C	64. D	96. D
30. C	65. C	97. B
31. B	66. A	98. C
32. C	67. B	99. C
33. A		100. C
34. A		
35. D		